Surviving the Unsurvivable

Natural Therapies for Cancer
A Revolutionary Integrative Approach

PAVEL I. YUTSIS, M.D.
with Stephanie Golden

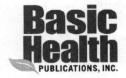
Basic Health
PUBLICATIONS, INC.

Basic Health Publications, Inc.
28812 Top of the World Drive
Laguna Beach, CA 92651
949-715-7327 • www.basichealthpub.com

Library of Congress Cataloging-in-Publication Data is available through the Library of Congress.

Yutsis, Pavel.
 Surviving the unsurvivable : natural therapies for cancer : a revolutionary integrative approach / Pavel I. Yutsis, M.D. with Stephanie Golden.
  pages cm
  Includes bibliographical references and index.
  ISBN 978-1-59120-302-5
 1. Cancer—Alternative treatment. 2. Naturopathy. I. Golden, Stephanie. II. Title.
  RC271.A62Y88   2012
  616.99'406—dc23

                                                2012038936

Editor: Roberta W. Waddell
Typesetting/Book design: Gary A. Rosenberg
Cover design: Mike Stromberg

Printed in the United States of America

10 9 8 7 6 5 4 3 2 1

Contents

- - - -

It's the Twenty-first Century—
Why Is Cancer Still with Us?

In Russia, where I first trained as a doctor, we didn't distinguish between conventional and alternative approaches to medicine. The expensive technological treatments common in the West were largely unavailable, so we had to explore other options. We used a wide range of less expensive, more accessible treatments, ranging from healthy diet, vitamins and supplements, herbs, and oxygen therapy to acupuncture and other forms of bodywork. We believed that whatever techniques worked to heal our patients were appropriate.

When I came to the U.S., however, I discovered that most of my American colleagues had no knowledge of these alternative treatments, and no interest in learning them. American medicine focused on new drugs and high-tech diagnostic and surgical techniques. While these techniques are often critically important, it's also a fact that *they have not improved overall survival from cancer.* A 2004 analysis of all studies done since 1990 of five-year survival rates after chemotherapy found that there has hardly been any progress at all in this regard.[1]

- In the U.S., chemotherapy improved the five-year survival rate from all types of cancer by only 2.1 percent.

- In the past twenty years, on average, lung cancer survival has increased by a mere two months.

- Chemotherapy for breast, colon, and head and neck cancers increased overall survival less than 5 percent.

One encouraging response to these discouraging facts is the recent growth of the field of integrative or complementary medicine, which combines conventional treatments—surgery, chemotherapy, and radiation—with alternative approaches, including some of those we used in Russia. Today, there is a new breed of cancer doctors you can turn to, and I wrote this book to make more people aware of who we are and what we can do to help cancer patients survive.

Two factors led me to undertake this book: first, my training as a Fellow in Integrative Cancer Therapy, which boosted my knowledge and enabled me to treat my patients more effectively; and second, the many challenges brought to me by patients who begged me to help them survive.

THE FELLOWSHIP IN INTEGRATIVE CANCER THERAPY

In 2010, Mark Rosenberg, M.D., pioneered the creation of the Fellowship in Integrative Cancer Therapy, under the auspices of the American Academy of Anti-Aging Medicine, an organization dedicated to educating physicians and the public about innovative science, research, and treatments that help people live longer. Dr. Rosenberg, who had long studied the effectiveness of chemotherapy, was prompted to create the Fellowship by several facts.

- Almost half his patients were likely to get cancer during their lives.

- Over half of all cancers can be prevented.

- Most cancer patients were already using alternative treatments with little, if any, guidance.

- Dr. Rosenberg also knew that only two-thirds of those with cancer survive more than five years, and he wanted to improve the odds.

The Fellowship organized the knowledge and experience of physicians around the world into a course whose graduates could offer improved cancer treatments that would extend people's lives, while also giving them better quality of life. These graduates, myself included, are integrative cancer specialists who use multiple methods—the ones you'll learn about in this book. We combine these therapies with surgery, chemotherapy, and radiation to make those traditional treatments more effective. Knowing all the current alternative therapies—some quite cutting-edge—that are available to you will make you more knowledgeable and empowered on the subject.

"I'M NOT A MAGICIAN—I'M A PHYSICIAN"

This is what I tell patients when they beg me to produce a miracle. No one can cure every case of cancer. But integrative cancer therapy certainly can make a difference, as the following four cases demonstrate. (In the following chapters you'll find detailed descriptions of all the treatments mentioned.)

Miriam

Miriam was diagnosed with uterine cancer and had a total hysterectomy. Three years later, a skin cancer on her face was removed. That same year, her doctor found that her cancer had metastasized to her lymph nodes. After undergoing more surgery, plus chemotherapy, Miriam, who was fifty-five, decided she wanted integrative treatment and came to me.

I started her on hydrogen peroxide, a form of oxygen therapy administered intravenously, in order to stop her cancer from progressing. She also had intravenous infusions of vitamin C and took a spectrum of supplements, including vitamin C by mouth, digestive enzymes, probiotics, high doses of vitamin D, and maitake D-fraction (an extract of an edible Japanese mushroom). While I was treating her, Miriam had three more surgeries to remove additional metastases in her colon. Then she had a colostomy. Finally her colon was removed, and she had twenty-four sessions of chemotherapy.

At this point Miriam's rabbi stepped in. Because the cancer had metastasized, he told her she should stop the alternative treatments and rely entirely on conventional medicine, which he believed worked better. Miriam decided to follow the rabbi's advice, even though her husband objected. "I disagree with your rabbi," I told Miriam, "but it's your body and your choice." She dropped my treatment and continued with chemotherapy. Although at first her condition improved, it soon deteriorated, and three years after she first came to see me, Miriam died.

I wanted Miriam to continue my treatments because I knew that conventional treatment is not effective for metastasized cancers. I can't say she would have survived with integrative treatment, but she'd have had a better chance. In any case, my treatment could have extended her life for a few years—and improved her quality of life. Unfortunately, I didn't have the opportunity to try and make that happen.

Sarah

Sarah, a seventy-one-year-old woman, knew me because her husband had consulted with me for possible treatment of colon cancer. After a short treatment, he decided he didn't believe in alternative therapies, stuck with conventional medicine, and eventually died from his cancer. Some time later, Sarah was diagnosed with B-cell lymphoma, a cancer that affects B-lymphocytes, a type of white blood cells. Having gone through the terrible experience of her husband's illness and death, she decided on integrative treatment and came to me.

Since I knew that chemotherapy has about a 50 percent success rate for her type of cancer, I suggested she include it as part of her treatment. But the chemo caused terrible side effects. Sarah became anemic and so weak she could barely move. She felt drained, she said, and begged for nutritional support. So I started her on intravenous infusions of vitamin C plus vitamin K, and on hydrogen peroxide therapy. I gave her multivitamins, turmeric (the yellow curry spice; it contains curcumin, a substance with known anti-cancer effects), high doses of coenzyme Q_{10} (CoQ_{10} is a substance found naturally in the body that boosts the immune system), Inflamma-Guard (an anti-inflammatory formula I developed), Onco-Guard (a formula of mine containing an antioxidant substance called sulforaphane), Immuno-Guard (an herbal formula that increases immune response), omega-3 fatty acids, and high doses of vitamin D.

Within two weeks Sarah felt much better. After she finished the chemo, she continued the alternative treatments, to which I added ozone therapy (another form of oxygen therapy). Her next PET/CT scan (a state-of-the-art imaging tool) revealed that her lymphoma had disappeared. As of this writing, Sarah has been free of cancer for two years.

Jessica

Jessica came to me as a forty-four-year-old mother of four who was absolutely determined to beat her advanced breast cancer and live to see her children grow up. She underwent every possible conventional treatment: lumpectomy, mastectomy with reconstructive surgery, and chemo (a three-drug cocktail known as CMF, plus tamoxifen).

Then Jessica learned that the cancer had metastasized to her left lung and the lymph nodes in her armpit. Her oncologist stopped the tamoxifen and gave her a new drug (an aromatase inhibitor) to lower the amount of estrogen in her body. But he also bluntly informed her there was nothing more he could do—her cancer was incurable.

Jessica refused to take no for an answer. "You wait and see," she told him. "I'll cure my cancer." She went off to Mexico for a one-month treatment with ozone, intravenous vitamins C and K, Coley fluid (also known as Coley's toxins, a mixture of killed bacteria that induces a strong immune response), and dendritic cell vaccine (a new form of immune therapy). Her next PET/CT scan showed no progression of the metastasis. Three months later, she returned to Mexico for another course of treatment. After that, she came to me.

I continued her vitamins C and K, and she self-administered the Coley fluid. She went on a special diet called the Gerson diet that stimulates the immune system, had coffee enemas, and took probiotics, oral vitamin C, selenium, omega-3 fatty acids, Inflamma-Guard, Onco-Guard, Immuno-Guard, and high doses of vitamin D, CoQ_{10}, and melatonin.

However, in spite of this extensive therapy, her next PET/CT scan showed some regrowth of the cancer. In response, I suggested insulin potentiation therapy (which uses insulin to boost the effectiveness of chemotherapy). That *stopped* the cancer, and as of this writing, there's been no further progression. I can't predict the future, but at the very least, alternative treatments extended Jessica's life for three years.

Jessica remains a great believer that she can fight her cancer—and I say, "Don't give up, Jessica."

Sheila

Sheila originally came to me for treatment of allergies, mental fogginess, and hypothyroidism (low-functioning thyroid gland). Six years later, she was diagnosed with breast cancer.

I started her on supplements, vitamin and oxygen infusions, and all the other treatments described above, plus extracts of graviola (soursop— a tropical tree with anti-cancer properties). I also suggested she have a lumpectomy to remove the tumor. "No way," she exclaimed. She also refused chemotherapy.

After two years on this regimen, tests for all cancer indicators were normal. Sheila continued all her therapies and kept to an anti-cancer diet. Five years later, she remains cancer-free.

MY MESSAGE TO YOU—INTEGRATION, MY FRIEND

These four patients illustrate four different attitudes toward treating cancer.

- Miriam tried integrative therapy, but went back to conventional treatment. Chemotherapy and surgery couldn't save her, and she died.

- Although Sarah chose alternative treatment, I integrated chemo into her regimen. Two years later, she was cancer free.

- Conventional treatment failed Jessica, so she turned to integrative therapy, which could not eradicate her cancer completely but did prolong her life by preventing it from progressing.

- Sheila insisted on alternative treatment only, refusing my advice to have a lumpectomy. Five years later, she's fine.

My experience treating these four—and many other patients—has taught me that the solution for maximizing cancer survival is *integration of treatment.* It means using *all* approaches: whatever is needed, whatever works to help the patient. That is precisely the philosophy of integrative cancer specialists, and I am proud to be one of them. Our number is growing and the Resources section will help you find one. With integrative treatment, you have not only a far greater chance of surviving cancer and extending your life, but a much better quality of life. In my vision, integration is the future of cancer treatment, and all of us—doctors and our patients—must work together to make that future bright. It offers your best chance to survive the unsurvivable.

Cancer and Its Multiple Connections

As preparation for learning about the many, varied cancer treatments in this book, it is essential to first read this very important review of ten cancer connections that allow the disease to gain an aggressive foothold in the body.

Often, when people hear the diagnosis *cancer* from a doctor, a chill goes down their spine. To them, that word spells a death sentence. Some are shocked and in a state of disbelief. Others feel angry and helpless; they wonder, "How can I survive this?" But all of them ask, "What is cancer, and what does it mean for me?"

That's a good question. The concept of what exactly cancer is has changed, which means that the whole approach to treatment has also changed. For many years, cancer was thought to be an infectious disease, caused primarily by a virus. As it turned out, that idea was wrong. If cancer were indeed an infectious disease, it would no longer be *the number two cause of death in the U.S.*[1] because there'd be a cure for it. Everyone would receive an anti-cancer vaccine (just like getting a swine flu vaccine during swine flu epidemics) and that would be that—cancer would be as rare as rubella. All over the world, vast sums have been devoted to attempts to develop such a vaccine, but without success. And no surprise there, cancer isn't infectious—period.

It's not primarily hereditary, either; only about 5 percent of all cancers are inherited. In order to understand and treat cancer effectively, you need to consider some new and different ideas about what it is and what causes it.

WE'RE LOSING THE WAR ON CANCER

It was in 1971 that President Nixon declared war on cancer, launching an intensive campaign to find a cure. Today, forty years later, the chances that an American will get cancer during his or her lifetime have actually *increased*. Between 1975 and 1977, for example, a man had a 33 percent chance of getting cancer. Between 2004 and 2006, that chance was up to 46 percent; and women experienced a similar increase.[2] What's more, the actual number of Americans who get cancer each year has increased as well, and this number has grown faster than the population as a whole. Between 1975 and 2006, the number of people who died from cancer did not grow—but neither did it decrease. And five-year survival of people with metastasized cancer is only a little bit higher than it was in 1970.[3] These sad statistics clearly show that cancer treatments have not been effective—at least not yet.

I believe that conventional medicine has failed to treat cancer successfully because its entire huge body of research and its rationale of treatment are based on incorrect, and perhaps incomplete, concepts of what cancer is and how it develops. In particular, conventional medicine has not recognized that multiple causes all operate together to produce the monster called cancer.

SO, WHAT IS CANCER?

Most oncologists agree that cancer is not a single entity but a conglomerate, characterized by *uncontrolled growth of normal cells, which develop the ability to invade other tissues of the body*. Almost all cancer cells are capable of initiating growth on their own, and they do not respond to signals telling them to stop. Unlike normal cells, they are not subject to the control mechanism of preprogrammed cell death (called *apoptosis*) that's necessary to keep the body functioning properly. Cancer cells' ability to grow is unlimited, and along the way they develop new blood vessels to bring them the nutrients they need to continue growing.

There are nearly 200 different types of cancer, but they all fall into three basic categories.

- *Carcinomas,* which arise in the skin and the endothelial tissue that lines and covers organs, blood vessels, and glands. Carcinomas include breast, lung, and colorectal cancer, among others.

- *Sarcomas,* cancers of connective tissue, including muscles and bones.

- *Leukemias and lymphomas,* cancers of the blood, bone marrow, and lymph nodes.

Not only is cancer not a single entity, *it's also not a simple, one-step event with a single cause.* It's a disease of the entire *system*—an extremely complex condition. For a cancer to develop, there must be a predisposition resulting from gene mutation, plus chronic environmental attack from such stressors as radiation, chemicals, unhealthy foods, free radicals (unstable atoms or molecule fragments that steal electrons from the molecules of body tissues in a destructive process called oxidation), electromagnetic fields, and many others.

HOW CANCER DEVELOPS

A case of cancer is the end product of a long process of development. It takes several decades before a mass of tissue appears that can be seen with the eye, felt by a doctor's hands, or observed on an x-ray, CT, or MRI scan. Cancer begins with genetic mutations that prevent the body from regulating the normal process of cell division, growth, and apoptosis. A mutation that damages either a gene that triggers growth, or a gene that slows or stops growth, can lead to uncontrolled growth—cancer. Such a mutated gene is known as an *oncogene.* There are over 100 known oncogenes, identified as causing different cancers. One, known as *bcr-abl,* is responsible for chronic myelocytic leukemia. Another, N-*myc,* causes neuroblastoma and small-cell lung cancer. While some people are born with a mutated, defective gene, most mutations result from long-term exposure to damaging environmental factors.

The body has a number of defense systems that protect against uncontrolled cell growth. The tumor-suppressor gene P53, for example, is part of a chain of events leading to the creation of a protein molecule that acts as a stop signal for cell division and prevents tumors from forming. P53 also promotes apoptosis—the event that cancer cells try desperately to avoid. The immune system also has a surveillance system of white blood cells that act as a kind of search-and-destroy mission attacking cancer cells. These defenses must be breached for cancer to develop.

The process of cancer development is called *carcinogenesis* or *oncogenesis*. It has three stages.

- *Initiation.* Cancer is initiated by an agent able to cause gene mutations that affect the growth-controlling mechanism. One mutation won't lead to cancer; that requires a number of mutations in a single cell, usually acquired over many years. That's why the risk of developing cancer increases with age. The older you are, the greater the chance that any given cell will develop enough mutations to turn into a cancer cell. When the cell becomes able to proliferate out of control, it enters the initiation phase of cancer.

- *Promotion.* The cell is now vulnerable to promoters, environmental agents that turn damaged cells into malignant cells. Alcohol, excess fat in the diet, nutrient deficiencies, and hormones, such as estrogen, progesterone, androgens, insulin-like growth factor 1 (IGF-1), somatostatin, and gonadotropin-releasing hormone (GnRH), can become promoters. Another promoter is *oxidative stress,* a term that refers to the destructive effects of free radicals (unpaired electrons). Promoters stimulate abnormal cell growth, damage tissue, or interfere with the body's protective mechanisms. At this point, cancer has appeared. But it may never grow into a tumor large enough to cause a problem.

- *Progression.* In this stage, the cancer has become large enough to be seen or felt, to cause such symptoms as pain or bleeding, or to be detected by a blood test, x-ray, or CT scan. Early-stage tumors are limited to one part of the body. But as they grow, they create new blood vessels to bring them the nutrients they need (a process called *angiogenesis*). They increase in size and begin to invade nearby tissues.

Overall, there are two basic elements that initiate cancer and further its development: *growth factors* and cancer's multiple connections. Growth factors are substances made by the body that regulate cell division and cell survival. Conventional oncology agrees that these, which include the following, are stimulating components in cancer development.

- *Insulin-like growth factor 1 (IGF-1)* is a protein similar to insulin that stimulates the growth of many types of cells. Higher than normal levels of IGF-1 may increase the risk of several types of cancer.

- *Epidermal growth factor (EGF)* is a protein made by many cells in the body and by some types of tumors. It causes cells to grow and differentiate (become more specialized).

- *Vascular endothelial growth factor (VEGF)* is a substance made by cells that stimulates angiogenesis (new blood-vessel formation).

- *Basic fibroblast growth factor (bFGF)*, which also promotes angiogenesis.

Cancer's multiple connections together constitute the second basic factor, and will be explored next.

CANCER'S MULTIPLE CONNECTIONS

As I've said, many factors come together to create the entity called cancer. I must emphasize that cancer is not a problem just limited to the breast, or the colon, or whatever part is affected. It's a whole-body disease, connected to lifestyle, diet, age, and the functioning of different body systems. You could say that cancer is well connected.

I've identified ten specific factors that play major roles in promoting carcinogenesis by making it possible for initiation, promotion, and progression of cancer to occur much more easily. I've named these factors the *cancer connections* because they create an environment in the body that allows cancer to become more aggressive and tougher to combat.

CONNECTION 1—THE GENETIC CONNECTION

In the past, hereditary factors were considered the most significant cause of cancer. It is now known, however, that this theory is not correct, and that relatively few cancers originate in inherited mutations. Between 5–10 percent of breast cancers are due to mutations in two genes called

"Why Me?" Asks Jack

Jack, who's been my patient since 1996, had quite a few health problems: allergies, hypothyroidism, and three different types of cancer—colon, prostate, and chronic leukocytic leukemia (a cancer of white blood cells). Over the years, I have treated him quite successfully with a combination of chemotherapy, vitamin C, and hydrogen-peroxide infusions, plus about thirty different herbs and vitamins. Jack's leukemia is in check, his PSA level is normal (PSA, or prostate-specific antigen, is a protein used to test for prostate cancer), and he shows no signs of colon cancer. But he still wants to know, "Why did I get those cancers?"

Why indeed? Jack is eighty-eight now. For many years, he's had a sweet tooth, so he eats a lot of cake, cookies, and candy. His triglycerides (a type of fat found in the blood) and cholesterol levels are always elevated. As this chapter explains, Jack has several cancer connections.

BRCA1 and BRCA2, whose functions include regulating cell growth and division and repairing damaged DNA. Mutations in the tumor-suppressor gene P53, the most frequently found genetic changes in all types of cancer, are also hereditary. Mutations in BRCA1, BRCA2, and P53 are passed down through families, and people who have them face an increased risk of developing cancer, since these genes are unable to play their roles in preventing unchecked cell growth.

Other types of cancer that appear to be caused by genetic changes are retinoblastoma of the eye, Wilms' tumor, and malignant melanoma. People with type A or AB blood (blood type is inherited) are also at a greater risk of developing cancer at some point in their lives. And an abnormal chromosome known as the Philadelphia (Ph) chromosome, created during cell division, contributes to the development of chronic myeloid leukemia.

In other cases, a gene may undergo changes that promote cancer development. For example, when oxygen levels in the tissues fall, a gene known as HIF-1 alpha is switched on, enabling cancer cells to survive by burning sugar (see Oxygen and Sugar Connections, following).

CONNECTION 2—
CANCER'S SWEETHEART, THE SUGAR CONNECTION

Cancer *loves* sugar. This is a really close connection that involves the way the body metabolizes carbohydrates. There are two basic types of carbohydrates, simple and complex. The term *sugar* refers to simple carbohydrates, small molecules that the body absorbs quickly. Examples are refined products, such as white flour and table sugar, or sucrose, which consists of a molecule of glucose and a molecule of fructose. Complex carbohydrates—starches, such as whole grains—are large molecules that take longer to be absorbed.

When you eat a carbohydrate, your digestive system breaks it down into small molecules so it can enter the bloodstream in the form of glucose. The pancreas responds to the higher level of glucose in the blood by secreting insulin, a hormone that enables the glucose to move into the cells, which break it down in a process called *glycolysis.*

Carbohydrates are essential nutrients, but a problem arises when people eat too many *refined* carbohydrates, especially table sugar and high-fructose corn syrup. All the cells in the body metabolize glucose, which is crucial for proper brain functioning, but fructose is metabolized by the liver. If you eat large amounts of sugar, the liver converts the fructose in the sugar molecule into fat. Scientists now believe that this deposit of fat in the liver causes *insulin resistance,* a condition in which the cells' normal response to insulin is reduced. To compensate, the pancreas secretes more insulin, but eventually, it cannot keep up with the body's need. Blood glucose rises, since the glucose is not being taken into the cells, and the result is diabetes, high cholesterol, high blood pressure, and high triglycerides—a group of risk factors together known as *metabolic syndrome* or *syndrome X.* People who are obese or diabetic or have metabolic syndrome are at higher risk for cancer.

Normal body cells do not rely exclusively on glucose to generate energy. They actually derive most of their energy from oxygen, in a process called *cellular respiration,* which follows glycolysis and occurs in tiny structures within the cell, called *mitochondria.* By contrast, cancer cells *cannot* use oxygen to generate energy; they live off sugar. In cancer cells, glycolysis occurs at a much higher rate than in normal cells. So it's not surprising that doctors use PET scans to detect cancer by showing the locations of sugar-burning cells in the body.

Researchers now suspect that insulin resistance, by triggering increased secretion of insulin, actually promotes the growth of tumors. (Endometrial cancer is one type that has been linked to high insulin levels.) Not only do the higher levels of insulin provide the glucose that cancer cells need in order to grow, but this extra insulin also provides a signal to the cells to metabolize more and more glucose. (That's why sugar is cancer's sweetheart.) Some cancers may actually need this growth signal in order to become malignant.

It makes a lot of sense, then, that an essential step for both preventing and treating cancer is to avoid sugar. Lowering the level of blood glucose deprives cancer cells of their basic nutrient, giving the immune system a boost in fighting the cancer. One study found that when volunteers were given high doses of glucose, sucrose, honey, and orange juice, their neutrophils (a type of white blood cell) actually lost some of their ability to neutralize invaders. That's why my treatment program starts with a low-sugar diet.

More important, avoiding sugar in the diet can sidestep the entire sugar connection and its consequences: fatty liver, insulin resistance, obesity, diabetes—all the steps along the path to cancer.

CONNECTION 3—OXYGEN, CANCER'S ENEMY

Cancer's sugar connection is intimately related to its oxygen connection. In fact, cellular respiration and glucose metabolism are like two siblings fighting for dominance in the family. To be healthy and function properly, normal cells and tissues must be well oxygenated. In fact, people whose oxygen utilization is sufficient will never develop any cancer in their life. Unfortunately, only about a third of the population breathes deeply enough to take in sufficient oxygen.

If a cell's oxygen supply becomes inadequate, it is likely to malfunction and switch to using glucose instead of oxygen as its fuel source. The process of extracting energy from glucose in the absence of oxygen is called *fermentation*. It's a primitive form of metabolism, common in undifferentiated (unspecialized) cells. As cells become cancerous, they actually regress to a more primitive, unspecialized form, in a process known as de-differentiation, and become capable of uncontrolled division and growth. This is carcinogenesis.

It was the German physician/scientist and Nobel laureate Otto Warburg who made this discovery about the metabolism of cancer cells during the 1920s. At around the same time, the Hungarian physician/ scientist Albert Szent-Györgyi, another Nobel laureate, observed that in cells undergoing malignant growth, insufficient oxygen is present. When cancerous tissue grows and generates energy without oxygen, far fewer free radicals are produced than normally. Although excessive free radicals are damaging, a certain number of free radicals are needed for normal body function. When too few free radicals are produced, nothing stimulates glucose to get involved in cellular respiration. As a result, glucose fermentation increases, producing a waste product called lactic acid that, in turn, creates an even more malignant environment in the cell. Because oxygen is absent, there is nothing to stop this process; it can go on forever.

In normal cells, the mitochondria are the furnace that burns oxygen to generate the large amounts of energy cells need. Mitochondria also play a role in regulating normal cell growth and death. But just like genes, they can be damaged by free radicals, thereby becoming unable to use oxygen effectively. New studies have connected cancer to defects in the mitochondria with the resulting oxygen deficiency in cells. Researchers discovered abnormalities in *cardiolipin,* a complex lipid (or fat) found in mitochondria that is essential to their function. Found in all tumors, these cardiolipin abnormalities severely impair the cell's capacity for cellular respiration. Other research has found that prostate tumors with reduced levels of oxygen are more virulent than those with normal or higher levels of oxygen.[4]

These discoveries highlight the drastic consequences when oxygen loses the family feud to sugar. They also suggest that bringing more oxygen to oxygen-deprived tissues can strengthen the immune system and even kill cancer cells, or at least make them less aggressive and slow the progression of the disease. This is why oxidative therapies are always a component of my anti-cancer treatment.

The struggle between oxygen and sugar is also relevant to the process of angiogenesis by which tumors create new blood vessels to bring them nutrients that enable them to grow. Some therapies you will read about in later chapters are designed to inhibit angiogenesis, on the principle that blocking it will prevent tumors from growing. However, there is a growing controversy regarding angiogenesis. The rationale for anti-angiogenesis is that it starves the cancer cell of glucose. But this treatment *also* starves the cell of oxygen, which is also transported through the blood—and at this point, no one knows if that's even worse. Right now, there's no way to determine whether new blood vessels bring more oxygen or more glucose to the cancer cell. It might turn out that cutting oxygen supplies to the tumor by inhibiting angiogenesis actually promotes its growth, because it then turns to burning sugar. Physicians are thus faced with a dilemma—to inhibit angiogenesis or not? I'll confront this dilemma throughout this book.

CONNECTION 4—THE PH CONNECTION

It's clear that cancer growth occurs in a low-oxygen environment. Such an environment is also acidic, meaning it has a lower pH than healthy, oxygenated cells, which are slightly alkaline. (The pH scale indicates the acidity or alkalinity of a tissue, from 0, strongly acidic, to 14, strongly alkaline. Normal blood pH ranges from 7.36 to 7.4.) There's a difference, however, between extracellular or intercellular pH (the pH of the space outside the cells) and intracellular pH (the level of acidity inside the cell wall). Cancer develops easily when the *extracellular* pH is acidic, because glycolysis produces large amounts of lactic acid as a waste product. This acidity actually promotes cancer development, through the following process.

- Lactic acid outside the cell causes a decrease in the cancer-killing activity of white blood cells.

- Acidic pH outside the cell facilitates production of substances that promote angiogenesis, enabling the cancer cell to supply itself with more and more glucose.

- Acidic pH makes it easier for the cancer cell to invade other tissues and metastasize.

If cancer thrives in a low-pH environment, it's logical that raising the pH can damage cancer cells. And indeed, researchers have found that administering alkaline substances intravenously can raise the extracellular pH of tumors, disrupting the chemical pathway by which glucose feeds cancer cells. The result: cancer-cell death. Cesium chloride, cesium and rubidium carbonate, sodium carbonate, and sodium bicarbonate have all been tried successfully as cancer treatments.

Chapter 7 discusses a novel approach to regulating pH that was developed by Mark Rosenberg, M.D. He found that increasing the level of lactic acid inside the cancer cell lowers the pH so much that the acid essentially burns the cell and destroys it.

CONNECTION 5—THE MID CONNECTION

MID stands for *metabolic immunodepression,* a change in metabolism that eventually depresses the immune function. Russian Professor Vladimir Dilman developed MID as a theory linking cancer to a disturbance in the way carbohydrates or fats are metabolized. MID helps you better understand cancer's connections with sugar, obesity, and aging.

According to Professor Dilman, MID is a depression of the immune system caused by the following chain of events.

- Consumption of excess simple (refined) carbohydrates leads to excess glucose in the blood, triggering the pancreas to secrete more insulin, which lowers blood glucose.

- Over time, insulin resistance develops, along with high insulin levels (hyperinsulinemia), which lower blood glucose (hypoglycemia).

- The body responds to low blood glucose by pulling fat out of fatty tissues in order to generate energy, increasing the level of free fatty acids and triglycerides in the blood.

- The result is elevated blood levels of LDL cholesterol (the bad kind).

- Cholesterol then accumulates in the membranes of crucial immune-system cells, particularly T lymphocytes, which attack cancer cells, and scavenger cells called macrophages, which gobble them up. The cell membranes become rigid and inflexible. The T lymphocytes cannot stimulate the growth of new T lymphocytes, so a shortage develops. The macrophages fail to do their job of engulfing and digesting cancer cells. At this point, MID has reached its final stage, and the immune system is severely depressed.

The process of immunodepression has two components—metabolic and immune—demonstrating the intimate connection between these two body systems.

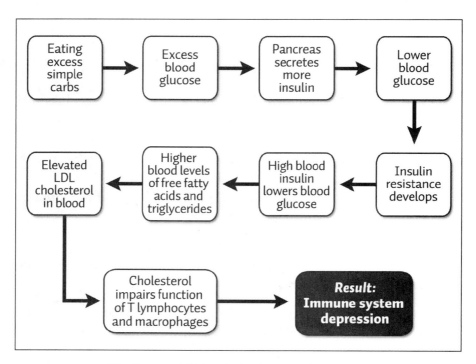

The Process of Metabolic Immunodepression

An Insulin Experiment

Professor Dilman performed this experiment with a group of women who had breast cancer. They had symptoms of insulin resistance, high blood levels of insulin, high LDL cholesterol and triglycerides, and low numbers of new lymphocytes—all of which indicated immunodepression. Dilman gave the women an insulin-lowering drug called phenformin (the older brother of metformin or Glucophage, which is widely used in the U.S. to treat type 2 diabetes), and after nine months found that all the abnormalities caused by MID had been reversed—and their production of lymphocytes was back to normal. He had restored the functioning of their immune systems.

In this experiment Dilman showed that it's possible to reverse the metabolic changes of MID and give the immune system a much better chance to fight off cancer. The beauty of MID is that it sets the stage for treatments that can both prevent the growth of cancer cells and help the immune system battle tumors already present.

CONNECTION 6—THE IMMUNE CONNECTION

Most physicians and researchers have known for decades that the immune system has an army of forces that can fight outside invaders, including cancer cells. The traditional idea was that the immune system protects everyone by distinguishing *self* from *nonself*. Anything recognized as *self* is accepted, and anything identified as *nonself*, or foreign—including cancer cells—is attacked by T lymphocytes and macrophages, just as in the MID model. Unfortunately, this theory hasn't helped to make cancer treatment more effective.

In the late 1990s, however, Polly Matzinger, a researcher at the National Institutes of Health, proposed what she called the Danger Model of immunity. The Danger Model suggests that the immune system reacts not to foreignness but to alarm signals sent by damaged tissues. Matzinger used this analogy: a community where the police accept anyone they already know, but kill all newcomers represents the self-nonself model. By contrast, she explained, "In the Danger Model, tourists and immigrants are accepted, until they start breaking windows." The police are the white blood cells. In the Danger Model, if newcomers do no harm, they're ignored.[5]

Matzinger's theory sets the stage for cancer treatments that activate immune defenses by stimulating the body to signal that something dangerous is happening—cancer. Chapter 5 describes these immunomodulation treatments, which use vaccines to stimulate the immune response.

CONNECTION 7—THE INFLAMMATION CONNECTION

Inflammation plays a major role in the development of cancer, since tissues that are chronically irritated can become malignant. Then the tumor itself accelerates the inflammatory process.

The great majority of cancer patients have proteins circulating in their blood that indicate the presence of inflammation in the body. These are known as inflammatory markers. Of great importance in the development of cancer are substances called cytokines, proteins that act as messengers of the immune system. Some, including tumor necrosis factor alpha and interleukins 1, 2, 6, and 8, promote inflammation, which is to say they attract immune cells to injured tissue. The enzymes cyclooxygenase (COX) and lipoxygenase (LOX) also contribute to inflammation. They are converted by arachidonic acid (a fatty acid) into pro-inflammatory molecules called eicosanoids, which include prostaglandins, thromboxanes, prostacyclins, and leukotrienes.

Another marker frequently used to test for inflammation is C-reactive protein, which is often elevated in cancer patients. An old-fashioned test for detecting inflammation is the erythrocyte sedimentation rate (ESR or sed rate); an extremely elevated ESR is one indicator for multiple myeloma, for example.

Any long-lasting inflammation in the body—arthritis, autoimmune diseases, fibromyalgia, or infections—can contribute to the development of cancer. Still another source of inflammation was first identified by Edward C. Rosenow, M.D., who for thirty years was head of experimental bacteriology for the Mayo Foundation. Rosenow came up with the concept of oral focal infection. Microorganisms from a localized infection in the teeth or gums, or sometimes the tonsils, can spread through the bloodstream, due to a mutation that enables them to exist in different forms depending on the conditions of their environment. Their spread can lead to a general inflammation throughout the body—which, in turn, can contribute to the development of cancer.

This means that a forgotten, untreated dental infection can spread to other parts of the body. So here is a simple way to help prevent cancer—take care of your teeth so you have no infections in either your teeth or your gums.

CONNECTION 8—THE OBESITY CONNECTION

There is not the slightest doubt that cancer is linked to obesity. In 2011, an analysis by the American Institute for Cancer Research found that about 100,500 cases of cancer each year are due to obesity.[6] Another study of 900,000 adults found that death rates were 42 percent higher for obese men compared to those of normal weight. For obese women, death rates were 88 percent higher.

In the previous section I explained the connection between cancer, obesity, and insulin resistance. Overweight causes cancer in other ways as well.

- Fatty tissue secretes estrogen. Higher blood levels of estrogen increase the risk for breast and endometrial cancer.

- Fatty tissue also increases the blood levels of other hormones, including testosterone and progesterone, which promote the growth of some kinds of cancers and prevent normal cell death.

- Obesity increases the risk for acid reflux, a condition in which the stomach contents leak back into the esophagus because the muscles that close off the bottom of the esophagus do not work properly. The reflux can damage the esophagus and eventually lead to esophageal cancer.

CANCERS LINKED TO OBESITY

▪ Breast	▪ Gallbladder	▪ Multiple myeloma
▪ Colorectal	▪ Kidney	▪ Pancreatic
▪ Endometrial	▪ Leukemia	▪ Prostate
▪ Esophageal	▪ Liver	

CONNECTION 9—THE TOXICITY CONNECTION

Toxins of all kinds are closely connected to cancer development. The toxicity connection is present in in every chronic degenerative disease, and cancer is no exception. This is so important that Chapter 9 is devoted entirely to this ninth connection.

CONNECTION 10—THE STRESS CONNECTION— CONNECTING ALL THE DOTS

Mental and emotional stress is a cancer connection that ties together all the others.

It is well known that traumatic life events—bereavement, divorce, job loss or insecurity, or the serious illness of a family member—evoke physiological responses in the body that can cause disease. In particular, research has shown a connection between stress and cancer. While some experts believe that single, short-term, severely stressful events are more important for triggering cancer development, I believe that chronic stress is much more of a contributing factor, because the body has a mechanism to cope with a single stress.

It is also important to recognize not only that mental and emotional stress is one of the cancer connections and a cause of cancer development, but that actually having the cancer is a severe stress in itself, with physical, social, and psychological effects. For those with cancer, the failure to properly address this source of stress can lead to deterioration in their condition.

Stress Connected to Sugar, Obesity, and MID

Chronic stress is a persistent presence that forces the human body to conserve energy, just as, during hot weather, utility companies ask customers to use their air conditioners less so there will be enough electricity to keep the whole system working. In the case of stress, conserving energy means the body uses less ATP than it should.

The molecule ATP (adenosine triphosphate) is the actual energy unit that's produced and stored in mitochondria through the processes of glycolysis and cellular respiration. Generating ATP from carbohydrates involves several processes.

- *Glycolysis,* which does not require oxygen. The rate of glycolysis in malignant cells is about 200 times higher than in normal cells. If there is insufficient oxygen present, the cell then uses fermentation to generate energy in the form of ATP. However the amount of energy conserved and stored in the cell through this pathway is far less than in the two following processes.

- If sufficient oxygen is present in the cell, cellular respiration begins with a process called the *Krebs cycle*. It is a series of enzymatic reactions that produce energy which can be used by every system of the body.

- Cellular respiration then continues with *oxidative phosphorylation*, which occurs in the mitochondria. This process moves electrons from electron-donor molecules to acceptor molecules and is the final step in producing ATP.

Even though the body under stress is conserving energy, the level of glucose in the blood remains high. This can be explained in terms of the hot-weather analogy, in which high temperatures represent the glucose level. You may be conserving energy by not running your air conditioner, but the temperature is still elevated. In the same way, conservation of energy by body cells doesn't bring the glucose level down—it stays high. And as a response, the insulin level goes up. Three events follow this, all associated with cancer connections.

- Obesity: Obesity connection
- Elevated glucose levels: Sugar connection
- MID: MID connection

Stress and the Inflammation and Immune Connections

Chronic stress destabilizes the body's natural repair mechanisms, which in time initiates an inflammatory process in the body (the *inflammatory connection*). Stress also induces malfunction of the immune system, and in this way it contributes to the *immune connection*.

Stress and the Oxygen and Genetic Connections

Now add to the network of stress connections the fact that cortisone and adrenalin, the hormones the body produces in response to stress, cause frequent vasoconstriction (narrowing of the blood vessels). In time, vasoconstriction leads to oxygen deficiency in the tissues (hypoxia) and . . . the *oxygen connection.*

And finally, chronic mental stress, by impairing the normal cell reproduction cycle, can cause gene mutation—which brings in the *genetic connection.*

You see, then, that cancer's great network of connections ties all the body systems to cancer's activity, thereby keeping them all in the family.

DETECTION AND DIAGNOSIS

A knowledge of cancer's connections helps in detecting it, since there are excellent diagnostic tests based on all of them. Genetic tests, imaging tools, and tumor markers are all techniques that help discover the presence or potential of cancer earlier, making it easier to treat.

Genetic Tests

The test for the BRCA1 and BRCA2 genes uses DNA analysis of a blood sample to discover whether a woman has a mutation in either gene that puts her at higher risk for breast cancer. There are also tests for HER1 and HER2, two other genes that, when mutated, promote breast-cancer growth, as well as for the growth-controlling gene P53.

Knowing the specific oncogene that is present in other cancers may be important for diagnosis and treatment.

Imaging Tests

Tests that create images revealing the presence of a tumor are more widely available than they used to be. MRI, CT, and PET scans and other types of imaging are good diagnostic modalities.

- *Magnetic resonance imaging (MRI) scan.* Creates detailed pictures using powerful magnets, radio waves, and a computer.

- *Computed tomography (CT) scan.* A series of detailed images of areas inside the body, taken from different angles, are created by a computer linked to an x-ray machine.

- *Positron emission tomography (PET) scan.* A small amount of radioactive glucose is injected into a vein, and a scanner is used to make detailed, computerized pictures of areas inside the body where the glucose is used. Because cancer cells gobble up more glucose than normal cells, the pictures can be used to find cancer cells in the body. (This is the sugar connection in action.)

- *PET/CT scan.* This new tool combines CT and PET. The PET scan images can help detect abnormalities in cellular activity, while the CT scan shows the size, shape, and location of a tumor.

- *Colonoscopy.* This procedure uses a thin, flexible tube with a video camera attached to examine the colon and rectum for early signs of colorectal cancer.

- *Mammography.* Most women are familiar with this x-ray of the breast. The question is, does it save lives? Many women with a history of breast cancer among their female relatives are advised to have regular mammograms beginning at age thirty-five. Unfortunately, most of these women have BRCA 1 and 2 mutations.

BRCA, as you may recall, is the gene that repairs DNA damaged by radiation. So a mammogram gives these women an extra dose of radiation when they already have a mutated gene that can't repair any damage. For this reason, I believe that a mammogram can harm these women much more than it can help them, especially since it can not only induce cancer, but can cause the most aggressive type. Many women with a strong family history of breast cancer who had routine early mammograms went on to develop very aggressive cancers and died within a year of diagnosis.

There's yet another problem with mammograms. The majority of women who receive their first one at age forty showing no cancer, then go on to have regular mammograms once a year, actually increase their chances for breast cancer from radiation exposure by an estimated 30 percent by the time they reach fifty (having a mammogram once every two years is just as bad). I believe it is far preferable to choose a breast sonogram or an MRI instead, neither of which involves radiation.

Tumor Markers

Tumor markers are substances produced either by tumor cells or by other body cells in response to the presence of tumor cells. Markers are found in blood or urine, in tumors, or in other tissues of the body. Most tumor markers are proteins, but some are genetic materials or other substances. These markers are used to detect cancer, to plan treatment, and to measure how patients respond to treatment. Table 1 below shows the most important tumor markers and those I use most commonly in my practice, with the types of cancer they're used for.

Determining estrogen and progesterone sensitivity (that is, whether these hormones stimulate tumor growth) is another very important test for breast cancer. Biopsied tissue is used to detect the tumor and whether it is sensitive to either estrogen or progesterone. The test also helps determine the stage of the cancer. The results are central in planning treatment.

TABLE 1. TUMOR MARKERS	
MARKER	TYPE OF CANCER
Alpha-fetoprotein (AFP)	Liver
Beta-HCG	Testicular and ovarian
CA 15-3	Breast
CA 27.29	Breast
CA 125	Ovarian
CA 72-4	Ovarian, pancreatic, stomach
CA 19-9	Colorectal, pancreatic
Carcinoembryonic antigen (CEA)	Colorectal, lung, breast
Human chorionic gonadotropin (HCG)	Testicular, ovarian
Prostate-specific antigen (PSA)	Prostate

FINAL THOUGHTS

While it is true that cancer can be detected earlier than it used to be, so far this advance has done nothing to significantly improve the chances for surviving it. That is why I have synthesized important concepts in integrative oncology, which have never before been brought together in this manner, into my theory of the *cancer connections*. These connections offer an updated model, which I hope will serve as a basis for integrative oncologists to design their treatments. I deeply hope, too, that my theory will enable many around the world to receive the treatment they so fervently desire and so desperately seek.

Surviving the unsurvivable is a long, tough, unpleasant journey. To beat the odds, you must travel this path to its successful conclusion with hope and passion, belief and desire, perseverance and determination. This book will provide the map for your journey. It will equip you with knowledge and understanding. The rest is up to you, your physician, and God. God bless you in this endeavor.

— — —

PART ONE

The Conventional Trio of Treatments

Physicians and scientists have different perspectives on the mass of tissue that is a cancer tumor. For my purposes here, I look at the tumor as a mass with two major components.

- The largest part of a tumor consists of its *bulk,* which is made up of pieces of necrotic (dead) tissue: dying cells and other waste materials.

- The *cancer stem cells* occupy only a minute part of the tumor but are by far its most important—and dangerous—component. These cells are what cancer treatment focuses on, and they play the major role in its success or failure.

Cancer stem cells are able to divide into other stem cells, which are malignant and can spread to other parts of the body, or into more differentiated daughter cells that stimulate proliferation (growth) of the tumor mass. Differentiated cells are more developed or mature and tend to grow and spread at a slower rate than undifferentiated tumor cells.

Cancer stem cells are extremely prolific, always ready, willing, and able to replicate, germinate, and produce millions of progeny. In the language of oncology, it is said that they enable the cancer to spread, proliferate, and metastasize.

In treating cancer, *both* the bulk of the tumor *and* its stem cells must be addressed. Reducing the size of the tumor is called *debulking,* and it is usually done using one or more of the conventional trio. Unfortunately, while these treatments destroy the bulk, they don't necessarily reach the stem cells. This is where problems can arise, for if the stem cells aren't destroyed, the cancer can and will grow back.

SOME CANCERS THAT FOLLOW THE CANCER STEM-CELL MODEL

- Acute myeloid leukemia
- Brain cancer
- Breast cancer

- Neuroblastoma
- Pancreatic cancer
- Testicular cancer

CHAPTER 1

— — — —

Surgery, Chemo, Radiation

*I*t took an entire army of CIA operatives, Defense Department forces, including specially trained Navy Seals, and a presidential executive decision to kill Osama Bin Laden. It will be much harder to eliminate advanced metastatic cancer, which is capable of being far smarter, more vicious, and more vigilant than even the most hated terrorist in the world. The three basic weapons in the arsenal for this assault are the conventional trio of surgery, chemo, and radiation.

SURGERY

Surgery is the oldest member of this treatment trio. As long ago as 1600 B.C., physicians of ancient Egypt cut tumors out with knives or red-hot irons. More recently, physicians believed that cancer spread from its original location to nearby lymph nodes and then to more distant parts of the body. The theory was that completely removing the original tumor would control the cancer. This did improve survival, but only to a certain point.

Most cancers continue to be treated first with surgery, which is the treatment of choice in two-thirds of all cases. Why is surgery so widely used? Because it removes the bulk, creating the impression that the entire tumor has been eliminated. In many cases that actually happens, but not always.

Today, the primary goal of cancer surgery is to completely eliminate the tumor and decrease the risk that it will recur or spread. Surgery may also be used preventively, to remove abnormal cells so they don't have a chance to become malignant, and to remove certain nonmalignant cancers. Cancer surgeons also perform diagnostic, preventive, reconstructive, and palliative procedures (which relieve symptoms, such as pain and pressure, but don't cure the cancer).

Diagnostic Procedures

Once cancer cells have been identified, a surgeon performs a biopsy to obtain tissue that can be analyzed to determine the precise nature of the cancer and its extent, or stage. *Staging* a cancer means determining its severity, based on its location, the size of the tumor, whether lymph nodes are involved, how abnormal the cells have become, and whether the tumor has metastasized.

- *Fine-needle aspiration* biopsy uses a thin, hollow needle, which is inserted into the tumor to collect cells that are then examined under a microscope.

- *Core needle biopsy* uses a larger needle that extracts fragments of tissue, which makes it possible to examine the cell structure of the tumor.

- *Cutaneous punch biopsy* uses a circular tool to take tissue samples from the full thickness of the skin, including its deeper layers.

- *Laparotomy* is an incision made in the abdomen so the surgeon can examine the interior. This procedure has been mostly replaced by laparoscopy but is still sometimes used to stage ovarian and some types of testicular cancer. (*Thoracotomy* is the equivalent procedure done in the chest.)

- *Laparoscopy* involves a small incision in the abdomen, through which the surgeon pumps gas that pushes the internal organs away from the abdominal wall. A laparoscope, a thin tube that holds a video camera, is inserted through the incision. The surgeon can see the area on a video screen and can insert instruments through the tube to take tissue samples for a biopsy. Laparoscopy is also used to surgically remove a tumor.

- *Lymphadenectomy* is surgical removal of lymph nodes, which are then examined for signs of cancer cells.

- *Sentinel lymph node mapping* is a procedure that finds the lymph nodes the cancer will most likely spread to first (that's why they're called sentinel nodes). A dye or a radioactive material is injected and it travels to the sentinel node. The node is removed and examined under a microscope.

- *Surgical biopsy* is done when the cancer cells are in a place that can't be accessed by a needle, or when a larger amount of tissue is needed. The surgeon uses a scalpel to remove a piece of the tumor (an incisional biopsy), or to remove the entire area of cancer cells.

Surgical Resection

Resection, or removal of the tumor, is the major type of cancer surgery. The surgeon plans the procedure by taking into account the location of the tumor, its stage, the patient's general health, and how the surgery is likely to affect her or him. Since the goal is to remove all the cancer cells, the surgeon may also need to resect parts of structures surrounding the tumor. The amount of tissue removed often depends on which organ is involved. For example, an entire lobe of the lung or liver is usually resected. Some cancers cannot be completely removed by surgery and may require additional radiation therapy.

Extensive surgery may stimulate an inflammatory process and thereby promote further growth of the cancer. The kinder and gentler the surgery is, the less inflammatory response it will produce, helping avoid further cancer progression. My advice is to find a surgeon who has a philosophy of restraint and wants to remove as little tissue as possible.

Advances in surgical techniques have enabled surgeons to perform reconstructive procedures at the same time as tumor removal in the breast, jaw, and genital areas. In these procedures, the surgeon transplants tissue from another area, such as the back or abdomen, to fill in areas where a large mass has been removed, restoring both form and function.

Newer Surgical Techniques

- *Cryotherapy* (or *cryosurgery*) uses a small probe at a very low temperature that is inserted into the tumor and kills cancer cells by freezing them. It may cure small tumors but is generally used as a palliative treatment.

- *Radiofrequency ablation* is used for liver cancer. A thin probe is inserted through the skin into the tumor and heated using high-frequency radio waves. The heat destroys the cancer cells.

- *Laser surgery* uses a beam of high-energy light to destroy cancer cells and is most often used to treat cancers on the surface of the body or the lining of internal organs. It's also a palliative measure that can shrink tumors obstructing the respiratory or digestive tract. It cannot, however, be used for invasive cancer.

- *Electrosurgery* uses a high-frequency electrical current sent through a wire to cut off cancerous tissue. One version is the LEEP (loop electrosurgical excision procedure), which uses a wire loop to remove pre-cancerous cells and noninvasive cancer from the cervix.

RADIATION

Radiation therapy uses different types of high-energy (ionizing) radiation to kill cancer cells by damaging their DNA. Radiation is used alone or in combination with surgery and/or chemotherapy to completely eliminate cancer. It can also be a palliative treatment to relieve pain. In the future, radiation may become a primary treatment for numerous cancers: bladder, brain, cervix, esophagus, larynx, lung, oral cavity, prostate, rectum, throat, and thyroid, as well as lymphomas, and for tumors elsewhere in the body that cannot be operated on because of their location.

The type of radiation used depends on the nature of the cancer and the size of the tumor. Radiation sources include the following.

- *High-energy photons.* Photons are bundles of energy—gamma rays or x-rays—that are emitted by a radioactive substance, such as cesium or cobalt 60, or produced by a machine called a linear accelerator. Gamma rays are higher-energy than x-rays.

- *Charged particles,* such as electrons, neutrons, or protons, are produced by a linear accelerator, which directs the beam of particles at the target tissue.

Radiation therapy can be applied either externally, by a machine outside the body, or internally, via radioactive material placed inside the body.

Treatment Planning

Careful planning makes it possible to decrease the damage radiation causes to normal tissues. Planning begins with simulation, using three-dimensional CT, MRI, or PET scans of the tumor and the surrounding tissues. The radiation oncologist uses sophisticated computers to determine the precise area to be treated, the amount of radiation the tumor will receive, how much of a dose the normal tissue near the tumor can receive, and the safest angles for delivering the radiation doses. Planning also includes methods to prevent organs that are particularly sensitive to radiation, such as the ovaries and testicles, from being irradiated.

External-Beam Radiation Therapy

External-beam photon or electron radiation is the most common form of radiation therapy. There are many different techniques for delivering it.

- *Three-dimensional conformal radiation therapy* uses MRI, CT, or PET scans with sophisticated computer software to map the tumor location in three dimensions. The radiation beams are delivered from several directions to very precisely shaped target areas to minimize radiation to normal tissue.

- *Intensity-modulated radiation therapy* is a new approach that uses computers to map the tumor in three dimensions, aim photon beams from different directions, and modulate the strength of the different beams.

- *Stereotactic radiation therapy* is an extremely precise technique that delivers a large dose of radiation to a small tumor without too much damage to normal tissue. It's used most often for brain and spinal cord tumors, but is being tested with other types of cancers as well.

The total dose of external radiation is usually divided into small fractions that are administered once a day, five days a week, for several weeks. Fractionating the dose makes it possible to give a high total dose more safely and effectively and to minimize damage to normal cells. Physicians are also experimenting with different delivery schedules.

- *Hyperfractionated doses* are smaller and are given more than once a day.

- *Accelerated fractionation* treatment gives larger doses daily or weekly to reduce the number of weeks of treatment.

- A *hypofractionation* schedule decreases the number of treatments by giving larger doses once a day or less often.

Internal Radiation Therapy

Internal radiation is also known as *brachytherapy,* which means short-distance treatment. Radioactive isotopes are sealed in containers—wires, pellets, capsules, or needles—that are implanted in or next to the tumor (*interstitial radiation*) or placed in a body cavity, such as the chest or rectum, near the tumor (*intracavitary radiation*).

Brachytherapy can deliver higher doses of radiation to a small area than external radiation, while causing less damage to normal tissues. Physicians sometimes use it in addition to external radiation to give extra radiation to a tumor without affecting normal tissue. It's given in either high or low doses and can be either temporary or permanent.

- In *high-dose-rate* brachytherapy, radioactive materials contained in hollow needles, fluid-filled balloons, or tubes, are placed in the area to be treated by remote control and then removed after about ten or twenty minutes.

- In *low-dose-rate* brachytherapy, the radioactive materials are left in place for one to seven days, then removed by the doctor. *Permanent brachytherapy* is a form of low-dose-rate treatment in which the radioactive substance is sealed in containers called *pellets* or *seeds* (the size of a grain of rice) that emit radiation for weeks or months. The pellets are left in place since they cause no discomfort or harm.

CHEMOTHERAPY

As applied to cancer, the term *chemotherapy* means treating cancer with chemicals. Alternate terms are *antineoplastic* (anti-cancer) and *cytotoxic* (cell-killing) therapy. Unlike radiation and surgery, which target specific areas, chemotherapy drugs travel through the entire body and can kill cancer cells that have spread. About 90 percent of all malignancies are treated with chemotherapy. There are over 100 different chemotherapy drugs, usually used in combinations of two or more to enhance their effectiveness. Through multiple mechanisms, these drugs can stop tumor cells from developing, multiplying, and spreading. Chemotherapy can cure some cancers and improve survival for others. In many cases, unfortunately, chemotherapy offers only relief from pain and discomfort (palliation).

Table 1.1 shows how chemotherapy affects different cancers. The source for this information dates back to 1988. I've purposely used this old data to make the point that not much has changed since then. The only difference is that it may now be possible to add testicular carcinoma to the list of curable cancers.

TABLE 1.1. EFFECT OF CHEMOTHERAPY ON DIFFERENT CANCERS

CURABLE	IMPROVES SURVIVAL	PALLIATION
Acute childhood lymphocytic leukemia	Acute adult lymphocytic leukemia	Adrenal carcinoma
Acute promyelocytic leukemia	Breast adenocarcinoma	Bladder carcinoma
Burkitt's tumor	Colorectal cancer	Brain tumors
Choriocarcinoma	Ewing's sarcoma	Chronic leukemias
Diffuse mixed and large-cell lymphoma	Hairy cell leukemia	Colorectal cancer
Hodgkin's lymphoma	Osteosarcoma	Endometrial carcinoma
	Small-cell lung carcinoma	Esophageal carcinoma
	Wilms' tumor	Kaposi's sarcoma
		Lymphocytic lymphoma
		Malignant melanoma
		Multiple myeloma
		Neck and head cancer
		Prostate cancer
		Soft-tissue sarcoma

Adapted from Wyngaarden, JB, and Smith, LH Jr, *Cecil Textbook of Medicine*, 18th ed. (Philadelphia: J.B. Saunders, 1988)

Both the way tumors grow and the variability in the way the drugs affect people influence the success or failure of chemotherapy.

Tumor Growth and the Cell Cycle

The speed and character of tumor growth is related to the *cell cycle* (the process by which the cell reproduces itself). This reproductive process has several phases.

- G0—the resting phase. Cells spend most of their existence in this phase, which can last a few years.

- G1—a growth phase.

- S—a synthesis phase, in which DNA is copied so the new cells will have exactly the same DNA as the parent cell.

- G2—continued growth and preparation for cell division.

- M—mitosis or cell division (the cell splits into two new cells).

The cell cycle is important because cancer drugs kill growing cells. They work by interfering with DNA synthesis in the S phase or with division in the M phase. Thus the number of individual cancer cells that are in a growing phase at the time of a treatment significantly affects how the whole tumor will respond. Since at any moment fewer than 10 percent of cells in a solid tumor are in the S phase, you can see why chemotherapy is not always very effective.

A tumor's rate of growth, or *growth kinetics,* indicates how rapidly its cells are replicating. The growth rate depends on three factors:

1. The proportion of actively dividing cells to the amount of growth factor present;

2. The doubling time (the time it takes for a cell to divide into two cells); and

3. The rate of cell loss.

The higher the growth rate, or activity of any of these factors, especially numbers 1 and 2, the more aggressive the cancer is and the less effective chemotherapy will be.

When a tumor becomes larger, its growth slows because of its increased demand for blood supply and oxygen. Large tumors contain a larger proportion of *nondividing* cells (the bulk) and are potentially less sensitive to chemotherapy, which mainly targets *dividing* cells. You might say that chemo drugs are not *interested* in killing these large tumors.

Pharmacogenomic Variability

Another factor influencing the results of chemotherapy is what's known as *pharmacogenomic variability.* This term refers to the fact that genetic differences among patients influence how their bodies respond to drugs. In other words, due to genetic predisposition, a person's individual cancer cells may be programmed to be sensitive to chemo drugs or, conversely, to not respond to them. Here is another instance of cancer's genetic connection.

Drug Combinations

Since the behavior of cancer cells is quite complex, chemotherapy works much better when several drugs are combined. There are several advantages of combination therapy over single-drug therapy.

- The combined action of the drugs is additive (their total effects equal their individual effects added together) or synergistic (the total effect is greater than the sum of their individual effects).

- Using drugs whose toxic effects don't overlap makes it possible to decrease the overall toxicity of the treatment. For example, a treatment can use three drugs that have lower toxicity than a single drug that might also be used for the same cancer. The combination treatment is more effective and less toxic for the patient.

- Combining drugs decreases resistance to each drug individually (see next section).

- Combination therapy improves the range of drug activity (that is, it makes the drugs more active).

TABLE 1.2. COMMON CHEMOTHERAPY DRUG COMBINATIONS

BEP	Bleomycin, etoposide, platinum (cisplatin)	Testicular
CMF	Cyclophosphamide, methotrexate, 5-FU	Breast
R-CHOP	Rituximab, cyclophosphamide, hydroxydaunorubicin, Oncovin (vincristine), prednisone	Hodgkin's lymphoma
CHOP	Cyclophosphamide, hydroxydaunorubicin, Oncovin (vincristine), prednisone	Non-Hodgkin's lymphoma
M-VAC	Methotrexate, vinblastin, doxorubicin, cisplatin	Bladder
VAD	Vincristine, Adriamycin (doxorubicin), dexamethosone	Multiple myeloma
ABVD	Adriamycin (doxorubicin), bleomycin, vinblastine, dacarbazine	Hodgkin's lymphoma
CAF	Cyclophosphamide, Adriamycin (doxorubicin), 5-FU	Breast
PVB	Platinum (cisplatin), vinblastine, bleomycin	Testicular
MOPP	Mustargen, Oncovin (vincristine), prednisone, procarbazine	Hodgkin's lymphoma
FOLFOX	5-FU, oxaliplatin, leucovorin	Colon

MDR: Multiple Drug Resistance

Cancer cells are smart, vicious, and vigilant. They can learn to resist cancer drugs, which can then no longer prevent them from growing and reproducing. This is a major problem in chemotherapy. In large tumors, chemotherapy can eliminate the most sensitive cells, while the rest become drug-resistant and remain untouchable.

Cells become resistant by being exposed to chemotherapy drugs. In many cases this explains why, in advanced cancers, a second round of treatment has little or no effect. Some important mechanisms through which *chemoresistance* occurs are:

- Mutated enzymes. Chemo drugs target enzymes that are vital for cell survival. When these enzymes mutate, the drugs no longer affect them.

- Targeted genes mutate, making them less sensitive to specific molecular inhibitors.

- Decreased drug activation. For different reasons, some chemo drugs lose their potency during therapy.

- Cancer cells do not die when they should because proteins, such as P53, that are supposed to trigger normal cell death, have mutated.

- Increased drug degradation (that is, the drug breaks down) because enzymes are present that metabolize it.

- Drug interaction. Some chemo agents actively interfere with one another, preventing them from having their intended effect.

- Enhanced DNA repair. This means that the cancer cell develops the ability to repair its DNA after the drug has damaged it.

Measuring Treatment Response

The success of chemotherapy is measured by looking at the state of the disease when treatment is complete, using a number of response criteria:

- The drug cannot get into certain parts of the body, such as the brain and testes, for example. Determining whether a tumor is in remission, shrinking, growing, and so on, enables doctors to define whether the disease is cured with a complete response, meaning the cancer has completely disappeared; whether there is only a partial response; or whether the tumor is stable or progressing.

- In hematological cancers (those that affect the blood, bone marrow, and lymph nodes), medical professionals investigate on the molecular level to see whether there is *molecular remission,* that is, a lack of disease activity in the bloodstream and bone marrow. Or they may conduct genetic and chromosomal studies of the bone marrow to determine whether there is *cytogenic remission (cytogenic* refers to chromosome abnormalities).

Adjuvant Chemotherapy

Adjuvant chemotherapy is given after primary treatment with one or more of the conventional trio, to increase the chances for survival.

Breast cancer. After surgery and possibly radiation, the oncologist may give adjuvant chemotherapy to kill any cancer cells that are left and may have spread.

- *Hormonal therapy* lowers the amount of estrogen in the body; breast cancer cells need estrogen to grow. One often-used drug is tamoxifen, which interferes with estrogen's activity. Another type of drugs called aromatase inhibitors prevent production of estrogen.

- *Trastuzumab* (Herceptin), a type of drug called a monoclonal antibody, targets cells that make too much of the protein HER-2.

- New drugs being used for adjuvant therapy include bevacizumab (Avastin), a monoclonal antibody that prevents angiogenesis by blocking the action of vascular endothelial growth factor. It is used in combination with drugs called taxanes.

- *CMF* and other forms of combination chemotherapy are also used for adjuvant therapy.

Colon cancer. Adjuvant therapy is used in stage III colon cancer after surgery. 5FU/LV is a combination of fluorouracil and leucovorin to which other drugs, including capecitabine and oxaliplatin, may be added.

Neoadjuvant Therapy

This type of chemotherapy is given before the primary therapy in order to shrink the size of the tumor. In breast cancer, neoadjuvant therapy can decrease the size of a tumor that otherwise could not be operated on and can make it possible to conserve the normal breast tissue. Oncologists use the patient's response to the drug combination given as an indication of whether the treatment as a whole will be successful.

Chemotherapy Side Effects

As I see it, there are six different types of side effects from chemotherapy.

- Suppression of bone marrow function, resulting in fewer red blood cells.

- Toxicity to cells in mucous membranes, often causing for example ulcers in the mouth.

- Toxicity to skin and hair follicles, causing rashes and baldness.

- Teratogenic effects, meaning harm to the fetus of a pregnant woman.

- Sterility.

- Immunosuppression (decreased immune system function).

TABLE 1.3. SIDE EFFECTS OF CHEMOTHERAPY DRUGS		
DRUG	**CANCER**	**MAJOR SIDE EFFECTS**
Aminoglutethimide	Prostate, breast	Depression of adrenal gland function, causing weakness, fatigue, and other symptoms; dizziness, rash
Anastrozole	Breast	Hot flashes
Bleomycin	Thyroid, ovarian, cervical, testicular	Scarring of lung tissue (pulmonary fibrosis), occasional bone marrow toxicity
Busulfan	Polycythemia vera, chronic myelogenous leukemia	Scarring of lung tissue
Carmustine/ lomustine	Brain	Low white blood cell count (leukopenia), low blood platelet count (thrombocytopenia), liver toxicity
Cisplatin	Ovarian, thyroid, head and neck, testicular, lung, cervical	Damage to inner ear (ototoxicity), severe kidney damage, mild bone marrow damage
Cyclophosphamide	Lymphomas and leukemias	Hair loss (alopecia), bladder irritation with urine in the blood (hemorrhagic cystitis)

DRUG	CANCER	MAJOR SIDE EFFECTS
Cytarabine	Leukemias	Bone marrow suppression, central nervous system damage, suppression of the immune system
Dactinomycin	Wilms' tumor	Liver damage
Daunorubicin/ doxorubicin	Breast, acute leukemia, Hodgkin's lymphoma, lung	Heart damage from daunorubicin
Etoposide	Testicular, lung	Bone marrow suppression
5-Fluorouacil	Breast, prostate, stomach, colon	Gastrointestinal damage, bone marrow suppression
Imatinib	Chronic myelogenous leukemia, gastrointestinal stromal tumors	Fluid retention
Irinotecan	Colon	Bone marrow suppression
Leuprolide	Breast, prostate	Hot flashes
Melphalan	Multiple myeloma	Bone marrow suppression
6-Mercaptopurine	Leukemias	Bone marrow suppression
Methotrexate	Choriocarcinoma, leukemias, Wilms' tumor	Liver damage, bone marrow suppression, ulceration of the digestive tract
Paclitaxel	Ovarian, breast	Bone marrow suppression
Procarbazine	Hodgkin's lymphoma	Damage to fetus, secondary tumors
Tamoxifen	Breast	Hot flashes, blood clots, stroke, uterine cancer
Trastuzumab	Breast	Fever and chills
Vinblastine	Lymphomas	Bone marrow suppression
Vincristine	Acute lymphocytic leukemia	Nerve damage, some bone marrow suppression

INTEGRATING CONVENTIONAL
THERAPIES

Since in many cases one conventional modality by itself is inadequate, oncologists commonly use different combinations of the conventional trio: radiation plus surgery, radiation plus chemotherapy, and all three together. For example, they may use radiation before surgery to eliminate cancer cells outside the area to be operated on and after surgery to eliminate any cells that may remain. They may use chemotherapy both before and during radiation treatment.

But the possibilities for combining the conventional trio go far beyond this. New research suggests that both radiation and chemotherapy can stimulate an immune system response. In particular, radiating a tumor triggers an immune response in the body that may be able to contribute to the success of the radiation treatment. Combining radiation with monoclonal antibodies is another promising approach. It seems that the radiation actually wakes up the immune system and teaches it how to respond effectively to the cancer.[1]

Other researchers have noted that low doses of some chemo drugs, including arabinoside, Adriamycin, and methotrexate, may sometimes produce immune-stimulating effects. The theory is that low-dose chemotherapy causes increased synthesis of one or more lymphokines (substances produced by white blood cells that are part of the immune response), such as interferons, interleukins, and tumor necrosis factor. The idea is that boosting the immune system in this way can make it more effective in fighting the cancer. In other words, these researchers are actually addressing cancer's immune connecton. To take another example, the newest group of drugs coming onto the market are the monoclonal antibodies (*see* Monoclonal Antibody Therapy in Chapter 5) —which work by acting on the immune system. So congrats to the immune connection.

Even in conventional oncology, therefore, integration is beginning to play an important role. In Chapter 3, I'll discuss another form of integration: combining chemo and radiation therapy with hyperthermia, the use of heat, to treat cancer.

FINAL THOUGHTS

In stage I or II cancers, surgery may be the only treatment needed. Radiation, on the other hand, is effective as a single modality in only a few types of cancer. The most exciting member of the conventional trio is chemotherapy. An explosion of information in the field of molecular oncology at the beginning of the twenty-first century has led to some important advances, offering hope for a new generation of chemotherapy agents that are highly specific for tumor cells. These drugs may also be less toxic to normal cells and produce fewer side effects.

However, although chemotherapy can and does kill cancer cells, it doesn't have a particularly good cure record. There are many reasons why it doesn't eliminate the majority of cancers.

- Cancer cells become resistant to chemo because only a low proportion of tumor cells are in the *S phase* of the cell cycle at the time of treatment.

- The cancer cells that were in the G0 (resting) phase during a treatment go through the cell cycle and produce new cancer cells between treatments, enabling the tumor to grow back. (The intervals between rounds of chemo are no shorter than three weeks.)

- The toxicity of the treatment prevents some patients from continuing.

- In some cases the drugs can't get to the cancer site.

- The drugs used are not specific enough to the cancer cells being targeted.

- Not enough cells are killed in each round of chemo. Even when patients receive maximal doses of drugs, a fraction of the tumor cells always survives.

- In brain cancer, the drugs are unable to cross the blood-brain barrier (a natural barrier that prevents many substances from entering brain tissues).

- Chemotherapy rarely reaches the cancer stem cells.

- Chemotherapy kills P53, the apoptosis-controlling gene, thereby helping cancer cells to live forever.

- Chemotherapy does not correct the abnormal physiology that allows cancer to develop. And it does not address the cancer connections.

Quite honestly, when I review all the info I've just given you, I get scared myself. It's a big mass of scientific mumbo-jumbo whose concepts can be difficult for anyone who isn't a medical expert to understand, even in nontechnical language. But believe me, reading it carefully is most definitely worth your while. It proves a seemingly contradictory point: that the conventional trio is both *useful* and *useless*.

Cancer patients are scared of many things. Some are frightened by cancer itself and its deadly verdict. Some see the conventional trio—especially chemo and radiation—as a pretty menacing prospect. Indeed, sometimes people with cancer wonder what will kill them first—the cancer itself or the chemo and radiation. That's a great question, perhaps the most important one for cancer survivors to consider as they make their decisions about treatment options.

Read all the scientific mumbo-jumbo in this chapter thoroughly. Read it more than once. Then return to this page and pay attention to what I'm going to say right now.

The standard conventional formula—cut it, zap it, and kill it— actually *won't* cut it.

By now you understand why: mainly because this strategy leaves the cancer stem cells intact. Let me repeat: *no one can treat metastatic cancer without taking care of the cancer stem cells.* It's that simple.

I suggest you adopt a slogan based on the one that candidate Bill Clinton made famous: "It's the connections, stupid!" Cancer is like the Mafia: it's surrounded by connections—the cancer connections, all ten of them. And chemo and radiation are not powerful enough to make an offer to cancer that it can't refuse. But there is hope that researchers will someday develop the cancer connections to the point where such an offer can be made, bringing everyone further along the road toward a cure.

CHAPTER 2

— — — — —

Reduce Side Effects
with Nutritional Strategies

Now that you have a good grasp of what the conventional trio can and cannot do, I want to explore a different avenue for surviving cancer: that of nutrition. One goal of integrative oncologists like myself is to address cancer physiology and the cancer connections for my patients who are already receiving the conventional trio of treatments. And one way this is done is to use nutritional strategies that support the efficacy of the trio and help ward off some of their terrible side effects.

The path of nutritional strategies is full of pleasant surprises: preventing and reducing the side effects of chemo and radiation, improving digestion, lifting fatigue, increasing energy levels, gaining lost pounds, and—by the way—providing better outcome and improved quality of life.

So you might think, *Hooray*. Nutrients are joining the conventional trio team. "Not so fast," says the medical oncologist confronted with a patient who wants to take supplements. This doctor is expressing a very common disagreement with the idea of combining conventional therapies, especially chemo and radiation, with nutritional supplements. Vitamins and antioxidants are subject to extremely critical scrutiny by conventional physicians.

Their objections may sound ridiculous. What could be wrong with eating oranges and berries—great sources of antioxidants—while undergoing chemo and radiation treatments? Here's the answer. The conventional oncology point of view is that physicians conducting these treatments should promote the idea of creating large forces of free radicals in the patient's body to destroy cancer cells. By eliminating these free radicals, antioxidants and vitamins supposedly prevent them from having this healing effect.

In my opinion, and that of many other integrative medicine specialists, by this logic, physicians should advise cancer patients to indulge in huge amounts of fast foods loaded with trans-fatty acids (a fantastic source of free radicals) in unlimited amounts. Let them eat hamburgers and cheeseburgers, and don't forget hot dogs. If chemotherapy worked mainly by generating free radicals, it should be possible to treat cancer with all sorts of substances that generate free radicals—high quantities of sugar, for example. But of course there are many reasons why people with cancer shouldn't do this, even if they love McDonald's.

TO ANTIOXIDIZE OR NOT TO ANTIOXIDIZE?

There is a great deal of scientific evidence that antioxidants are highly effective. They:

- Improve the effectiveness of chemotherapy;

- May kill cancer cells;

- Protect normal cells;

- Decrease the toxicity of chemo and its side effects; and (most remarkably)

- Don't interfere with the therapy.

More than 300 studies have been published reporting on the use of antioxidants during cancer therapy. In fifteen trials with human subjects, over 3,500 patients survived longer when they took antioxidants while receiving conventional treatments.

Here are some examples of clinical studies that support antioxidant use during chemo and radiation. In a 2004 study of children with acute lymphoblastic leukemia, done at Columbia University in New York, researchers found that low intakes of antioxidants were linked with more negative side effects from chemotherapy. On the other hand, higher antioxidant intakes were linked with fewer therapy delays, much less toxicity, and a lower incidence of infection. Other researchers studied the antioxidant glutathione in combination with the chemo drug oxaliplatin for treatment of advanced colorectal cancer. They concluded that repeated glutathione injections protected patients from the side effects of oxaliplatin yet did not reduce the effectiveness of the drug.[1]

Another study, from 2005, looked at the effect of high oral doses of vitamins C and E plus beta-carotene used together with chemotherapy for patients with stages III and IV non-small-cell lung cancer. This study did not support the conventional belief that antioxidants interfere with the effects of treatment. In a 2003 study of 100 patients with metastatic lung cancer who were treated with chemo in combination with mela-tonin, patients who got the melatonin had a much higher survival rate.[2]

Doctors at the Institute for Biomedical Research at the University of Texas, Austin, found an improved survival rate in patients with lung, colon, and prostate cancer who received antioxidants. Researchers in Denmark gave vitamins C and E with selenium and essential fatty acids, plus coenzyme Q_{10} (CoQ_{10}), to thirty-two high-risk advanced breast cancer patients. Six of the thirty-two had partial tumor regression, and all thirty-two reported improvement in quality of life. None had metastases. Finally, a study done at Simone Protective Cancer Institute in Lawrenceville, NJ, and in Italy at the University of Cagliari came out with identical conclusions.

WHAT DO ANTIOXIDANTS ACTUALLY DO TO CANCER CELLS?

A hundred different studies have demonstrated that as chemotherapy proceeds, antioxidant levels drop. In fact, chemotherapy lowers antioxi-dant levels. And don't forget that cancer patients usually have low levels of antioxidants even before chemotherapy begins.

Having read the Prologue, you know that cancer cells are acidic due to increased lactic acid production (the pH connection). In an acidic environment, antioxidants become pro-oxidants—that is, they *create* free radicals, and therefore can be used as *targeted natural chemotherapy.*

Studies published in the *Journal of the American College of Nutrition* in 1992 and 1999 suggested that a high intake of antioxidants can damage cancer cells—and at the same time *protect* healthy cells. In fact, cancer cells can accumulate extremely high levels of antioxidants, while healthy cells cannot. Another interesting discovery is that antioxidants stimulate the immune system. Very high levels of antioxidants in cancer cells produce a series of reactions within these cells that prevent them from functioning and actually kill them.

So you see why integrative physicians often combine antioxidants with chemo and radiation therapy.

BENEFITS OF ANTIOXIDANTS DURING RADIATION THERAPY

Antioxidants can make radiation therapy more effective and reduce side effects, including:

- Blood count changes
- Eating problems
- Fatigue

- Hair loss
- Skin problems

For common antioxidants used with radiation therapy, see the inset on the following page.

BENEFITS OF ANTIOXIDANTS DURING CHEMOTHERAPY

Antioxidants—either prescribed by physicians or taken by patients according to their own programs—help reduce a wide range of toxic effects of chemotherapy:

- Bone marrow depression
- Cachexia (weight loss and weakness)
- Cardiotoxicity (heart damage)
- Hair loss

- Liver and kidney damage
- Lung damage
- Nerve damage
- Oral sores

For common dosages of antioxidants used with chemotherapy, see Table 2.1 on page 50.

ANTIOXIDANTS USED WITH RADIATION THERAPY

Vitamin A and carotenoids

- Improves effectiveness of radiation therapy
- Enhances immune response
- Makes cancer cells more sensitive to radiation
- Reduces toxicity to normal cells

Vitamin C

- Increased response to radiation treatment
- Reduced side effects

Vitamin E succinate

- Reduces damage in normal cells and therefore decreases side effects
- May increase damage to chromosomes in cancer cells
- In one study, reversed fibrosis (scarring and hardening of tissue) resulting from radiation

Glutathione

- Reduces side effects, making patients more likely to complete radiation therapy
- Probably does not interfere with radiation

CoEnzyme Q$_{10}$

- A mouse study showed reduced side effects of radiation

Selenium

- Prevents selenium depletion, which makes the body more sensitive to radiation

Melatonin

- One study showed fewer side effects and increased survival

ANTIOXIDANTS USED WITH CHEMOTHERAPY

Vitamin A and carotenoids

- May kill cancer cells while reducing toxicity for normal cells
- In head and neck cancers, one study showed better survival with fewer side effects
- High doses of vitamin A may damage organs, and high doses are associated with osteoporosis

Vitamin C

- There is no evidence suggesting that vitamin C makes chemotherapy less effective
- Some evidence suggests that vitamin C might make chemotherapy more effective
- In one study, combining vitamin C with doxorubicin reduced heart damage and was associated with improved survival

Vitamin E succinate

- Strong anti-cancer activity
- Protects healthy cells without interfering with chemo treatment
- Improved effectiveness of doxorubicin and cisplatin

Selenium

- When used with cisplatin, decreases toxic effect of drug on kidneys while increasing the drug's anti-cancer activity
- In one study, patients who took selenium with cisplatin had higher white blood cell count

Coenzyme Q_{10} (CoQ_{10})

- Combined with doxorubicin and trastuzumab to counteract heart damage

- In one study of patients with leukemia and lymphoma, protected heart function during chemotherapy
- Improves antitumor effect of doxorubicin
- Reduces mouth inflammation and diarrhea
- CoQ_{10} deficiency can lead to cachexia

N-acetylcysteine (NAC)

- Protects against hematuria (blood in the urine) resulting from chemotherapy with ifosfamide
- Since it may decrease effectiveness of chemotherapy, should probably not be used

Flavonoids

- Quercetin (from berries, apples, red onions, and yellow vegetables) enhances the effects of busulfan and cisplatin
- Quercetin may increase concentration of doxorubicin in the cell
- Tangeretin (from tangerines and citrus fruits) may reduce the activity of tamoxifen

Melatonin

- In human studies, increased survival, decreased nerve damage, brought platelets to normal level, decreased bone marrow suppression, and reduced cachexia

Green tea extract

- Enhances effectiveness of the chemo drugs from the anthracycline group without making them more toxic
- Reduces heart damage from doxorubicin
- Increases cancer-prevention effect of tamoxifen
- May enhance antiangiogenic activity of trastuzumab

TABLE 2.1. COMMON DOSAGES OF ANTIOXIDANTS FOR CANCER PATIENTS

Antioxidant	Dosage
Vitamin A	40,000–100,000 IU per day
Vitamin C	3,000 IU/(up to 125g per day in IV treatments)
Vitamin E	400–800 IU per day
Selenium	400 mcg per day (low dose)
CoQ$_{10}$	500–1,000 mg per day
Melatonin	Up to 20 mg per day
Resveratrol	10–500 mg per day
Quercetin	500–1,000 mg per day
Curcumin	500–1,500 mg per day
Green tea extract	500–1,000 mg per day
Whole foods antioxidants	10–12 servings of fruits and vegetables per day

NUTRITIONAL SUPPLEMENTS AND CHEMOTHERAPY

Several clinical studies have reported that combining nutritional supplements with chemotherapy improved the effectiveness of the treatment. There are many such combinations, which I've listed below.

It's hard to explain why so many physicians who treat cancer do not use these supplements. Their patients continue to experience all the difficulties of chemotherapy and never get the benefits that supplements can offer. Over the years, my patients have done much better when they followed my advice and applied the information in this chapter to their treatment plans. So please: pay attention!

As you read through the lists below, you may notice that the dosages I provide are different from dosages you've read elsewhere. That's because there's no standard protocol for supplements. My dosages are based on what has worked for my patients. I recommend that you follow them. These dosages won't give you any side effects.

You'll also notice that for some supplements, I give a wide range of dosages. Start at the lower level and work your way up. If you can tolerate a dose level and you feel ok, go higher.

Breast Cancer Studies

The following supplements were combined with doxorubicin/Adriamycin in treating breast cancer:

- Fish oil concentrate 2,500 mg containing EPA 900 mg, DHA 650, 1 capsule 3 times per day

- Genistein 40–60 mg per day

- Glutathione 60–600 mg per day

- Grape seed polyphenol 50–200 mg per day

- Green tea polyphenols (EGCG) 700 mg per day

- Melatonin 20–40 mg per day

- Quercetin 500 mg 3 times per day

- Red clover capsules 430 mg 2–3 times per day

- Rutin and other flavonoids 500 mg 3 times per day

- Selenium 400 mcg per day (maximum dose)

- Silymarin 500 mg 3 times per day

- Silymarin as silbinin 100–900 mg per day

Colon Cancer Studies

These supplements were combined with 5-fluorouracil to treat colon cancer.

- Avemar (fermented wheat germ extract) 1 packet (5.53 g) per day

- Curcumin 500–4,000 mg per day

- D-glucarate 50–1,000 mg per day

- Fish oil concentrate 2,500 mg (containing EPA 900 mg and DHA 650), 1 capsule 3 times per day

- Green tea polyphenols 700 mg per day

- Genistein 100–110 mg per day

- Glutamine 500–1,000 mg per day

- N-acetylcysteine 600–1,800 mg per day

- Vitamin D_3 3,000–5,000 IU per day

Lung Cancer Studies

Combined with carboplatin (Paraplatin)

- Beta-carotene (vitamin A) 10,000–40,000 IU per day
- Vitamin C 2,000–4,000 mg per day
- Melatonin 40 mg per day
- Vitamin E 400–800 IU per day

Combined with cisplatin (Platinol)

- American ginseng 200-1,000 mg per day
- Astragalus decoction 10–20 mg per day
- Genistein 100–110 mg per day
- Melatonin 20 mg per day
- Omega-3 fatty acids (DHA)
- Quercetin 200–1,200 mg per day
- Vitamin D 200–1,000 IU per day
- Vitamin K 45–500 mcg per day

Combined with cyclophosphamide (Cytoxan, Neosar)

- American ginseng 200–1,000 mg per day
- Genistein 100–1,100 mg per day

Combined with docetaxel (taxotere)

- Genistein 100–1,100 mg per day

Prostate Cancer Studies

Combined with cisplatin (Platinol)

- Genistein 100–110 mg per day
- Melatonin 1–20 mg per day
- Silymarin as silibinin 100–900 mg per day

Combined with carboplatin (Paraplatin)

- Silymarin as silibinin 100–900 mg per day

Combined with paclitaxel (Taxol, Onxol, Abraxane)

- Curcumin 500–4,000 mg per day
- Green tea polyphenols 700 mg per day
- Melatonin 1–20 mg per day

Lymphoma Studies

Combined with cyclophosphamide (Cytoxan, Neosar)

- Methylselenic acid (MSA)/ methylselenocysteine 200 mcg per day
- Sulfoethyl glucan 100–500 mg per day

Combined with doxorubicin (Adriamycin)

- CoQ$_{10}$ 100–600 mg per day
- Vitamin B$_6$ 50–200 mg per day

SPECIFIC BENEFICIAL SUPPLEMENT–CHEMO DRUG COMBINATIONS

Certain supplements have specific beneficial effects when combined with certain drugs. So I urge you to pay attention to the essential information that follows.

- DHA combined with paclitaxel makes it sixty-one times more effective and significantly less toxic. This means the patient can tolerate a dose that is over four times higher. DHA also reduced hair loss, nerve damage, nausea, and vomiting. Overall, patients had a better quality of life.

- GLA (an omega-6 fatty acid) increased the effectiveness of tamoxifen for breast cancer and of dexamethasone for leukemia.

- D-fraction maitake mushroom combined with cyclophosphamide resulted in 94 percent reduction in tumors, compared to 57 percent when the drug was given by itself. This supplement also reduced infections and side effects, including nausea and vomiting, hair loss, low white blood cell count, and pain.

- Genistein combined with cisplatin increased the absorption of the drug by cancer cells.

Avoid These Combinations

A few supplement-drug combinations should be avoided during chemotherapy.

- Beta-carotene with 5-fluorouracil

- Capsaicin (extract of chili peppers) with cisplatin or paciltaxel

- Glutathione during any chemo

- NAC with cisplatin or doxorubicin

- Tangeretin with tamoxifen

NUTRITIONAL SUPPLEMENTS AND RADIATION

Nutritional supplements can increase the effectiveness of radiation therapy in a variety of ways.

- In one study, beta-carotene increased survival and the effectiveness of radiation. It has been shown to protect the spleen. Beta-carotene is especially effective combined with niacinamide and is apparently more effective than vitamin A. *It should be avoided by lung cancer patients.*

- Vitamin B_3 (as niacinamide) dilates blood vessels, increasing blood flow in cancers that have developed a large blood vessel network. It creates high oxygen levels in cancer cells, making them more sensitive to radiation. (As you may recall, in the Prologue I described the dilemma over whether or not to prevent angiogenesis, pointing out that increasing the blood flow in tumors isn't necessarily a bad thing. With vitamin B_3, increasing blood flow looks like a great thing.)

- COX-1 inhibitors (arthritis drugs) and COX-2 inhibitors (including NSAIDs, which are pharmaceuticals, curcumin, and flavonoids, which are natural COX-1 as well as COX-2 inhibitors) make cancer cells more sensitive to radiation while protecting healthy cells. COX-2 inhibitors also prevent growth and metastasis of cancer cells. Start taking them two to three weeks before therapy begins.

- Resveratrol makes cancer cells more susceptible to radiation while protecting normal cells. Start before radiation begins.

- Mushroom extract (containing beta-1,3-glucan) protects immune cells in particular from radiation and stimulates the immune system. It protects bone marrow and prevents infections after radiation.

- Ashwagandha (Indian ginseng) protects healthy cells, increases white blood cell count, and increases blood-forming cells in bone marrow.

- Ginkgo biloba contains antioxidants and prevents DNA damage in healthy cells. It reduces metastasis by protecting blood vessel walls and is an anticoagulant, protecting against the higher risk of blood clots in cancer patients.

FIGHTING SPECIFIC SIDE EFFECTS OF CHEMO AND RADIATION

Nutritional supplements don't just work synergistically with chemo and radiation—they offer many other benefits as well. Nutrition is regularly used to counter particular problems caused by chemo and radiation therapy.

Three-quarters of cancer patients experience fatigue, stress, nausea and vomiting, and poor appetite, and as a result they eat badly and are poorly nourished. Yet only a third of these patients actually tell their doctor about these side effects. You should definitely let the doctor know about them, since nutritional supplements can help you feel a great deal better.

Fatigue

Some chemo drugs cause fatigue by damaging the mitochondria, which are in charge of producing energy. These supplements can boost your energy:

- Acetyl-L-carnitine 250 mg twice per day

- CoQ_{10} 100 mg three times per day

- Lipoic acid 100 mg twice per day

- Multivitamins including vitamin C and B vitamins

Cachexia

About half of those with cancer experience weakness and weight loss, which is a major cause of morbidity (sickness) and death. Weight loss results from stress, loss of appetite, and often from a higher metabolism rate caused by the cancer. In addition, the treatment itself may interfere with absorption of nutrients. Inflammation is related to cachexia, so nutrients that reduce cytokines, the proteins that promote inflammation, are used. The following nutrients might help.

- Flavonoids (including curcumin, grape seed extract, hesperidin, lacto-ferrin, pycnogenol [pine bark extract], and quercetin) 300 mg twice per day
- Omega-3 fatty acids, EPA/DHA, up to 18g per day
- Vitamin E 400–800 IU

These nutrients are used to build muscle:

- Egg whites
- Medium-chain triglyceride (MCT) oils (e.g., coconut) 1 tbsp. on full stomach
- Protein bars that contain a mixture of whey, soy, and rice proteins. Make sure you buy bars sweetened with stevia, not sugar in any form.

Nausea, Vomiting, and Aversion to Food

A number of chemo drugs cause nausea because they stimulate an area in the brain that controls vomiting. They also irritate the mucous lining of the stomach. These drugs include Adriamycin, cisplatin, darcarbazine, daunorubicin, 5-FU, high-dose Ara C, mechlorethamine, L-asparigni-nase, and strepozocin.

You can minimize nausea and vomiting by doing the following.

- Avoiding greasy, spicy, and acidic food
- Drinking vegetable juices to counter acidity
- Eating smaller portions more frequently instead of full-size meals

- Soothing your stomach with deglycyrrhizinated licorice root (DGL), gamma-oryzanol (rice bran oil), ginger extract, L-glutamine powder (4g dissolved in water or vegetable juice), marshmallow root, and slippery elm

These same supplements will help against food aversion, which many undergoing chemo develop. Start taking them several weeks before your first chemo treatment. Another tip: Don't eat your favorite food just before getting chemo.

Hair Loss

To minimize hair loss, wash your hair only every two days, avoiding harsh shampoos, especially any containing sodium lauryl sulfate. Air-dry it or use only the low-heat setting on your hair dryer.

- Antioxidants will protect the hair follicle and help your hair grow back faster and healthier.
- Curcumin 500 mg three times per day
- Decaffeinated green tea extract 100 mg three times per day
- Hesperidin 500 mg three times per day
- Quercetin 500 mg three times per day
- Vitamin E succinate 400 IU three times per day

Add a multivitamin and biotin (3 mg twice per day during chemo, then once per day) to this regimen.

Sore Mouth and Throat

Ulcer sores and inflammation in the mouth are painful, prevent swallowing, and result in dehydration and malnutrition. The sores may bleed.
  To minimize these side effects, do the following.

- Add 4g L-glutamine in 4 ounces of distilled water, swish in the mouth, and swallow one or two times per day. (Do not use in cases of brain tumor.)

- Don't consume hot, spicy foods and drinks.

- Don't drink alcohol or smoke.

- Don't use a mouthwash containing peroxide, fluoride, alchohol, or any other strong chemicals.

- Use a compounded (specially mixed) mouthwash containing grape-seed extract and stevia. One teaspoon is added to 4 ounces of distilled water. This mixture is antifungal, antibacterial, and antiparasitic, and it soothes an inflamed mouth and throat. You can swallow it.

- Use CoQ_{10} to protect the gums. Mix 100 mg of it with 1 tablespoon extra-virgin olive oil and swish the mixture in your mouth. Also use a toothpaste containing CoQ_{10}.

- Use a soft toothbrush.

Cardiotoxicity

Many chemo drugs cause toxicity that affects the heart; in fact this is one of the major causes of death related to chemotherapy. Heart failure can occur not only during the treatment but years later. The amount of injury to the heart usually depends on *how high the dose of drug was.* The damage may be permanent.

Chemo drugs that cause heart damage include actinomycin D, clophosphamide, cytarabine, daunomycin, doxorubicin, 5-FU, herceptin (which can cause severe heart damage and heart failure, plus strokes), mitoxantrone, Taxol, and taxotere.

A number of nutrients are great protectors against heart damage.

- Acetyl-L-carnitine 500 mg three times per day on empty stomach, in the form of L-carnitine fumarate

- CoQ_{10} 200 mg four times per day, starting one week before treatment and continuing for three weeks, then 100 mg three times per day. Doxorubicin lowers CoQ_{10} levels, making CoQ_{10} an important supplement, for it protects against both acute and delayed heart damage, decreases irregular heartbeat, and reduces free radicals.

- Curcumin 500 mg three times per day

- Decaffeinated green tea extract 100 mg once per day

- Flavonoid complex with quercetin, rutin, hesperidin: 250–500 mg of each, three times per day

- Hawthorne extract 500 mg twice per day

- Magnesium citrate 150 mg once per day

- Omega-3 fatty acids (2,500 mg [containing EPA 900 mg and DHA 650], one capsule three times per day) reduce irregular heartbeat, improve the flow of blood to the heart, and improve the function of the heart muscle.

- Propolis extract 400 mg twice per day

- Selenium can protect against heart damage from doxorubicin. A high dose of 800 mcg four times per day is needed, but since this dosage can be toxic, do not take it for longer than eight days during chemotherapy. A low dose of 200 mcg twice per day can be taken one week before treatment and continued one week afterward.

- Vitamin C (500 mg three times per day) protects against heart damage caused by doxorubicin. It may also increase the effectiveness of doxorubicin and other chemo drugs.

- Vitamin E succinate (400 IU, three times per day) given just before treatment can reduce acute heart damage, but not delayed heart failure. It does not reduce the effectiveness of doxorubicin.

Intestinal Problems

Chemo and radiation therapy can cause a variety of intestinal side effects, including diarrhea, dysbiosis (disturbance in the intestinal flora), immune reactions that result in food allergies, irritation of the mucous lining of the intestines, leaky gut syndrome (damage to intestinal lining that allows undigested toxins to leak into the bloodstream), poor absorption of nutrients, and yeast infections.

Nutrients that protect the gut include:

- Digestive enzymes (except when there are ulcers)

- L-glutamine (4g dissolved in 4 ounces distilled water, once or twice a day). Do not use in cases of brain tumor.

- Prebiotics: fructo-oligosaccharides (FOS) are plant sugars that promote growth of beneficial bacteria in the gut. They're used as a sweetener sprinkled on food. For dose, follow directions on the bottle.

- Probiotics, including lactobacillus and bifidobacterium

Bone Marrow Depression

A frequent cause of delay or outright discontinuation of chemotherapy is bone marrow depression. Nearly a third of patients need a lower dose for this reason. In addition, when patients with bone marrow depression need blood transfusions or blood-stimulating medication, over half develop nausea, and a quarter experience fatigue. But a variety of nutrients can protect the bone marrow.

- Curcumin 500 mg three times per day

- Folate 800 mcg once per day

- Methylcobalamin (vitamin B_{12}) under the tongue, 1 mg three times per day and twice a day when chemotherapy ends

- Multivitamins (without methionine)

- Vitamin B_3 500 mg twice per day

- Vitamin B_6 50 mg once per day

- Vitamin C 500 mg three times per day

- Vitamin E succinate 400 IU three times per day

Liver Damage

Because the liver works to detoxify the body from chemotherapy drugs and also to clear dead cancer cells, liver damage is common. Combining more drugs increases the risk. Taxol is particularly damaging to the liver. Liver-protecting nutrients include:

- Curcumin 500 mg three times per day

- D-glucarate 200 mg four times per day (can go up to 3g per day)
- Indole-3-carbole 200 mg three times per day
- Methylsulfonylmethane (MSM) 1–4g per day
- Milk thistle 400 mg twice per day
- Taurine up to 4g three times per day

Lung Damage

Busulfan causes fibrosis in the lung that can be acute or occur as long as ten years after chemotherapy. Combining chemo and radiation therapy increases the risk of lung damage, which is caused by free radicals. Several nutrients can protect the lungs.

- Bioflavonoid complex including quercetin, rutin, and hesperidin—for dose, follow directions on the product you're using
- Boswellia 300 mg twice per day
- Curcumin 500 mg three times per day
- Green tea extract 300 mg three times per day
- Vitamin E succinate 400 IU three times per day

Nerve Damage

Most chemo drugs aren't supposed to cross the blood-brain barrier, but this may happen when there is brain tumor, fever, high blood pressure, or neurological disease; when radiation therapy is targeted at the head; when a person is older; or when chemotherapy lasts a long time.

Nearly a third of patients treated with cisplatin suffer from polyneuropathy, or damage to nerves throughout the body. This drug also can cause tinnitus or hearing loss. Procarbazine can lead to ataxia (lack of muscle coordination), brain damage causing sleepiness, and confusion. These side effects may be acute or delayed. Nutrients that protect the nervous system include:

- Alpha-lipoic acid 200 mg twice per day

- CoQ_{10} 100–200 mg three times per day

- Curcumin 500 mg three times per day

- Ginkgo biloba 160–320 mg once per day on an empty stomach

- Magnesium ascorbate 750 mg three times per day

- Magnesium citramate 300 mg three times per day

- Milk thistle 175 mg once per day

- Quercetin 500 mg three times per day

- Vitamin E succinate 400 IU three times per day

Radionecrosis

Radiation damage to normal tissues is cumulative, and fractionating the therapy over several weeks can reduce this damage. Hard surfaces such as bone or implants can scatter the beam so that cells distant from the site being radiated can be affected, though to a lesser degree. Radiation injury can be acute, in the form of burns, or delayed, in the form of fibrosis or another cancer.

Tissues with cells that are particularly sensitive or are dividing fast are especially at risk for radiation injury. These include the bone marrow, the brain, the lymphatic system, the mucous lining of the stomach and intestines, and the spleen.

Certain people are also at higher risk for radiation injury:

- Older people

- Patients who have had both chemo and radiation

- People who eat few fruits and vegetables

- Smokers

- Those who eat a lot of red meat

- Those who have had frequent x-rays, including mammograms and CT scans

- Those with chronic disease, including diabetes and autoimmune disease

- Those with high iron and copper levels

- Those with poor nutrition

- Those under chronic stress (and this includes all cancer patients)

Two nutrients can protect cells from radiation injury:

- Alpha lipoic acid 200 mg twice per day;

- Ashwagandha (Indian ginseng) 5 cc of a 1:2 extract in water twice per day—this nutrient protects the cell's integrity and its DNA and protects the bone marrow, even increasing the number of bone-marrow cells after treatment.

FINAL THOUGHTS

What do people with cancer believe in regard to taking all these nutrients? A study of 760 people with breast cancer revealed that they took beta-carotene, selenium, and vitamins C and E during their chemo and radiation treatments. Over 60 percent took antioxidants overall. Thirty-nine percent took them during chemotherapy, 42 percent during radiation, and 62 percent while using tamoxifen. Remarkably enough, 69 percent took higher than normal doses of antioxidants. Clearly, the use of antioxidants among cancer patients is quite common.

Other sources too show that 69 percent of cancer patients take antioxidants during their treatments. In fact, over 80 percent of patients going to the famous MD Anderson Cancer Center in Houston used supplements, including antioxidants. Most did not have these prescribed by their doctors, but took them on their own.

Certainly research studies to document the effects of nutritional supplements are important and necessary. But these people with cancer have been taking supplements for years, and they feel much better. The naysayers will attribute these successes to the placebo effect. But I say that if a person takes specific supplements for a specific health problem connected to a specific cancer, and they relieve that problem, this is not a placebo effect.

So my advice to naysaying physicians is, even though the literature suggests that anti-cancer nutrients harm people with cancer and decrease the efficacy of chemo and/or radiation—and even though you believe they are no more than placebos, do not harm your patients by telling them not to take these supplements. The evidence for this position is virtually nonexistent. In fact, most studies show that nutritional supplements have a beneficial effect. Some show no effect, but none show a harmful effect. What's more, antioxidants have another benefit as direct cancer-killing agents— given in extremely high doses to cancer patients, many of them act as prooxidants and are therefore chemotherapuetic in nature. Even further, a large body of evidence indicates that antioxidants not only improve the efficacy of radiation treatments, but also protect normal cells in the surrounding tissues *and* decrease unpleasant side effects.

Most people who have cancer are pretty miserable. They're often fatigued and nauseated, they're getting bald, and they have diarrhea. If you're feeling this way, taking all the nutrients and supplements I'm advising may seem too exhausting and cumbersome to contemplate. But believe me, taking them is extremely important and will make a huge difference for you. If you feel you simply can't take dozens of tablets and capsules a day, then prioritize. Choose just those nutrients that are most relevant to your symptoms and your treatment goals.

Speak with others who have cancer, go to support-group meetings, and participate in online support forums to find out what other people's experience of supplements has been. If you're taking only conventional treatments, consider consulting an integrative physician, naturopath, or nutritionist. Most people with cancer don't hesitate to get second or third opinions from other oncologists, but seeking another opinion from an integrative physician can make you a real winner. Many who have consulted such doctors remain survivors to this day.

- - -

PART TWO

Powerful and Safe Integrative and Alternative Treatments

I've collected so much information about integrative and alternative cancer treatments that it's tough to decide where to start in describing it. But I want passionately to share it with you, so here goes.

But first, as you read, and later when you're making decisions about treatment, always keep in mind that if your physician, a friend, or a family member disagrees with what I tell you here, even if that person laughs at it or expresses very negative feelings on the subject, *it doesn't matter*. Don't let that person's response determine your choices. It's your life, and ultimately it's up to you to decide whether and how to use the information in this book. I urge you to educate yourself as much as you can. Do your best to accumulate all the information you think necessary. Speak with other cancer survivors who have been helped by an integrative/alternative approach; they will be more than happy to share their experience with you.

For an online forum, try the Best Answer for Cancer Foundation's Patient Survivor Center, www.bestanswerforcancer.org/patientsurvivor-center

Don't get discouraged, and don't allow anyone to knock you down with a statement like, "There's nothing we can do for you, but don't try any alternative treatments—they're just a waste of time and money." Simply go on learning in your own way. It is never a waste of anything.

In Part Two you'll learn about non-conventional therapies, modalities, techniques, and research directed toward the treatment of cancer itself and all the problems associated with it. Most of this information has been known for quite some time. Some of it is unknown—brand new, and maybe earth-shattering. But all of it is tremendously useful for anyone with cancer, and may even save your life.

I can only imagine how much more information, knowledge, and experience there would be if just a tenth of the money spent on research and development of chemotherapy were devoted to research on alternative treatments. But it's better to stop dreaming and focus on reality, which you'll discover in these pages.

CHAPTER 3

- - - - -

Why Alternative Therapies Work

Alternative therapies work because they address the cancer connections.

In the next section you'll read the story of my patient Barbara—a sad tale, yet also quite educational and even encouraging. Perhaps you'll be infected with the same passionate determination as Barbara and her son Alex, so that, as Alex put it, you'll want to "fight this sucker" with all you've got. Barbara's story will also show you the magnitude and diversity of the integrative arsenal. There is, in fact, a huge variety of alternative treatments that have been known for years, even decades. Others have come into use only recently among just a few health practitioners around the world.

It's also important to understand that no two integrative physicians will treat the same patient in exactly the same way. In the integrative/alternative world, there are no equivalents to standard chemo combinations like CHOP and MOPP. While integrative doctors do use some common, familiar combinations, such as vitamin C together with vitamin K, that's about it. Alternative physicians can choose among many different treatment combinations, and *all of them will be right*. At the same time, the basic rationale for alternative treatment protocols always remains a common denominator.

Alternative therapies are multifaceted. Some are quite simple, others quite complex. Some are inexpensive, others costly. Part Two describes those that alternative physicians consider most important, and which can be gotten now or possibly offered in the future.

- All nutritional supplements

- Cancer vaccines

- Carnivora (Venus flytrap)

- Detoxification

- Diet

- DMSO (dimethylsulfoxide)

- Escozine (extract of blue scorpion venom)

- Hyperthermia

- Insulin Potentiation Therapy–Low Dose(IPT-LD) chemotherapy

- Intravenous (IV) vitamin C

- Iscador (mistletoe)

- IV sodium bicarbonate

- Laetrile/amygdalin/B_{17} therapy

- Off-label use of drugs

- Oxidative therapies (hydrogen peroxide therapy, ozone therapy, hyperbaric oxygen therapy, ultraviolet radiation of blood or UVIB)

- Positive psychological/spiritual reinforcement

- Salicinium (homeopathic remedy)

- Stress-relieving techniques

- Thymus

- Ukrain (celandine)

This chapter discusses a number of these treatments; the rest are covered in the chapters that follow. To introduce you to the world of integrative/alternative treatment, though, I'll start with Barbara's story.

BARBARA'S ODYSSEY THROUGH ALTERNATIVE CANCER CARE

Barbara, a kind, quiet sixty-year-old woman, was diagnosed with advanced stage IV estrogen- and progesterone-positive breast cancer about four years before she came to see me. Because her cancer was so aggressive, her doctors at the time gave her just a year to live.

Before receiving this terrible prediction, Barbara had suffered the tragic loss of her husband. She also had some other health and lifestyle factors that an integrative physician would consider significant. She had multiple mercury fillings in her mouth (mercury is toxic, and leaks into the system from the fillings) and chronic infected root canals in two teeth. Habitually sleep deprived, she ate an extremely poor diet, heavy on such sweets as donuts and cookies, sugar, carbohydrates, and other junk food. After her husband's death, she began to work extremely long hours.

Very unfortunately, Barbara's surgeon could not remove her cancer mass because the tumor was so closely attached to her rib cage. He could only partially separate it from the rib cage and insert draining tubes to prevent fluid buildup in her chest. So the mass got larger and larger, producing many metastatic nodules (small lumps) around it. At this point, Barbara consulted a naturopathic physician, who started her on a number of naturopathic therapies, including multiple supplements. She had her mercury fillings removed and her two infected teeth extracted, and began detoxification with herbs, supplements, and diet. Banishing sweets, carbohydrates, junk food, and red meat from her diet, she ate large amounts of raw vegetables, whole grains, and some fruit.

Her thirty-two-year-old son, Alex, decided to devote his life to one goal: "To keep my mom around as long as possible." He used all his savings and took out several loans to take his mother to Italy, where she was treated by Dr. Tullio Simoncini, a prominent alternative physician, and the developer of IV sodium bicarbonate treatment, which changes the body's pH.

After that, Barbara and Alex visited cancer clinics in Mexico, where she was given a combination of high doses of IV vitamin C, IV vitamin B_{17}/laetrile, and IV DMSO; total body hyperthermia; and two cancer vaccines (Coley fluid and dendritic cell vaccine). (You'll find descriptions of these treatments below and in the following chapters.) After two courses of these treatments, Barbara's health improved dramatically. She felt much better, and to Alex it seemed she was almost in remission.

Barbara, Alex, and his fiancée Donna, who had also gone to Mexico, were all delighted, and Barbara convinced the others to travel to another Mexican city to visit a famous church. Leaving the church, they ate lunch in a neighborhood restaurant, then took a cab to their hotel. In the cab they were abducted by a Mexican gang that kidnapped people and killed them for their organs. The gang members stole their money and terrorized them for several hours. In the end they survived only because Barbara passed out and the frightened abductors threw them out of the cab as it passed through an abandoned area in the middle of nowhere.

It took several months before Barbara, Alex, and Donna recovered psychologically from this ordeal, and during this time Barbara's health spiraled downward. Her tumor markers, which had shown great improvement, deteriorated. Donna felt she could no longer deal with the complicated situation around Barbara's illness and left Alex. Barbara became depressed and withdrawn, but Alex remained determined to "fight Mom's cancer." His passion woke up Barbara's desire to survive.

They returned to Mexico for two more rounds of treatment, during which Barbara developed a pleural effusion (buildup of fluid between the layers of the pleura, a thin tissue that lines the lungs and the inside of the chest cavity)—a common mischief caused by cancer. Her lungs were tapped twice to drain the fluid. In her fourth round of treatment, Barbara received IPT-LD (low-dose, targeted chemotherapy strengthened by the addition of insulin), along with IV DMSO and high doses of IV vitamin C. Her doctors chose the chemo drugs for Barbara's IPT treatments using two different blood tests to determine the cancer's sensitivity to drugs. One blood sample went to the Research Genetic Cancer Centre in Greece, the other to Germany for the Biofocus test. (*See* Chapter 4.)

When she returned to the U.S., Barbara continued the IPT treatments and was also given Arimidex (anastrazole, an aromatase inhibitor that prevents estrogen production). During this period, fluid had to be drained from her lungs again. Her condition fluctuated—she would improve, then deteriorate.

Then Barbara got a new treatment, escozine, an extract of blue scorpion venom. In four months, her tumor markers improved significantly. For example, the breast cancer marker CA 15-3 dropped from 447.3 to 43.8 (normal limits, 7.5–53), and the metastatic breast-cancer marker CA 27.29 dropped from 743.5 to 10 (normal limits, 0–38.5)

Barbara continued IPT for another year, along with escozine, ozone therapy, and DMSO. But then a followup CT scan revealed metastases and small pathological bone fractures in her spine and pelvis. So the drug Zometa, which treats bone damage caused by cancer, was added to her regimen. She also began receiving local irradiation of the bone lesions. Her doctors (including myself) were thinking about trying salicinium, a new supplement that fools cancer cells into thinking that it is sugar, when Alex ran out of money. Nevertheless Barbara's relentless struggle to survive has continued.

I chose to elaborate on Barbara's case because of her seemingly miraculous survival, way past the dire predictions of her original doctors—all thanks to those alternative treatments. Cases like Barbara's abound, and it's in your best interest to disregard anyone who pooh-poohs alternative treatments.

THE VITAMIN C STORY

The story of vitamin C also describes seemingly miraculous healing. Vitamin C is one of the most common forms of alternative cancer treatment, and for good reason. It prevents cancer-cell proliferation, induces cancer-cell apoptosis, strengthens the immune system, and works well with other therapies, both conventional and alternative. It improves quality of life and—last but not least—it addresses quite a few of the cancer connections:

- Oxygen
- Inflammation
- Immune
- Sugar
- MID
- Genetic

Addressing the Oxygen Connection

Ascorbic acid has two types of anti-cancer effects related to the oxygen connection, and administered intravenously, it can act as either an antioxidant or a pro-oxidant, depending on the dose.

- Doses under 50g function as antioxidants, neutralizing free radicals and protecting healthy cells.

- Doses over 50g and up to 125g have a strong pro-oxidant effect. This is because ascorbic acid produces molecules of hydrogen peroxide (H_2O_2), an action that's significant because malignant cells are deficient in the enzyme catalase, whose function is to convert H_2O_2 into oxygen and water. Without the action of catalase, H_2O_2 builds up and creates free radicals that kill the malignant cells. Thus nontoxic vitamin C can destroy cancer cells just like many chemo drugs—and therefore it can and should be used as a chemotherapeutic drug.

Addressing the Inflammation Connection

High doses of IV vitamin C inhibit *inflammatory mediators* (cancer-causing substances that promote inflammation), including cytokines and prostaglandins. Ascorbic acid also inhibits COX-2, an inflammation-promoting enzyme. Breaking the chain of inflammatory reactions leads to a decrease in cancer aggressiveness and slows further progression of the cancer.

Addressing the Immune Connection

Accumulating in white blood cells, ascorbic acid becomes a commander-in-chief of the immune defense forces against viruses, bacteria, fungi, and tumor cells. It increases production of lymphocytes, which produce antibodies that improve immune function.

What's more, vitamin C increases production of interferon, a protein that prevents viruses from reproducing themselves—quite useful since cancer patients have poor immune function, so they frequently get bacterial and viral infections. This infection-fighting ability of vitamin C is well known among those with cancer, even those who choose only conventional treatment.

Addressing the Sugar Connection

Ascorbate (AA) and dehydroascorbate (DHA) molecules are different forms of vitamin C that are very similar to molecules of glucose and some other sugars. These vitamin C molecules can therefore *fool* cancer cells, which consume them instead of sugar and starve as a result. Ascorbic acid also causes a reduction in the cancer promoter IGF-1 (insulin-like growth factor 1).

Once, years ago, I checked a patient's sugar level with a glucose meter after giving him a high dose of vitamin C and was astounded to find that his sugar was over 400. Then I realized what had happened. Ascorbic acid could not only fool the cancer cells—it had fooled the glucose meter.

Addressing the MID Connection

Ascorbic acid's resemblance to sugar enables it to prevent or reverse the whole process of metabolic immunodepression, which starts with excess blood glucose. Ascorbic acid fools not just the cancer cells but the entire body into thinking that it's sugar. As the body takes in ascorbic acid instead of sugar, the actual blood sugar drops. With decreasing sugar levels comes a decrease in blood cholesterol and triglyceride levels, followed by lower cholesterol levels in T-lymphocytes. T-lymphocyte function improves considerably, which in turn boosts the function of the entire immune system.

Addressing the Genetic Connection

The gene HIF-1 alpha is usually activated when oxygen levels in a cell fall, enabling these cells to survive by means of glycolysis. According to several animal experiments, suppression of this gene is linked to retarding tumor growth. Other research shows that overexpression (expression means *switching on,* and overexpression means *hyperfunctioning*) of this gene is associated with a higher death rate of cancer patients. Researchers found that high-dose IV vitamin C prevented the overexpression of the gene, which meant that the cancer cells could not generate the energy they needed to live on.[1]

Vitamin C's Safety and Efficacy Are Well Established

A number of laboratory and clinical studies have proven the great safety and effectiveness of high doses of vitamin C. In the late 1970s, the chemist and Nobel Prize laureate Dr. Linus Pauling teamed up with Dr. Ewan Cameron to research the role of vitamin C in treating cancer. They administered it both orally and intravenously to people with terminal disease. The results were impressive. A group treated with IV vitamin C survived 300 days longer, on average, than an untreated group. Twenty-two percent of those treated with high-dose vitamin C survived for several years after the treatment ended, compared with only 0.4 percent of the control group. A 1976 study of 100 patients treated with ascorbic acid and 1,000 control patients, and a 1978 study of 294 patients treated with ascorbic acid and 1,532 control patients, both found that survival time in the treated patients was at least two to four times longer than in the control groups—and the treated patients had a much better quality of life.

I can't talk about vitamin C treatment of cancer without mentioning Dr. Hugh D. Riordan, who founded the Center for the Improvement of Human Functioning International (now called the Riordan Clinic). He came up with the idea for the RECNAC project (RECNAC = *CANCER* spelled backward), whose goal was to discover why cancer develops and how to treat it without damaging normal tissue. In one RECNAC study, twenty-four terminal cancer patients received between 10g and 60g of intravenous sodium ascorbate (a form of vitamin C) for eight weeks. No complications or side effects resulted. This study proved without a doubt that high doses of vitamin C are safe.

I'll cite two more studies further proving this point. In one, conducted in Japan in 1982 by Dr. A. Murata, fifty-five terminally ill patients received 5–30g of vitamin C daily; they survived 246 days. By comparison, fourty-four control patients survived for only 43 days.[2] In the other, from 2005, scientists at the National Institutes of Health reported that ascorbic acid killed cancer cells while leaving normal cells unaffected.[3]

The fact is that hundreds of alternative/integrative physicians around the world have been using vitamin C as an anti-cancer treatment for years. The best current thinking suggests administering it intravenously combined with vitamin K, in a ratio of 100 (C) to 1 (K) for the greatest synergistic effect. Clinicians have also noticed that vitamin C IV therapy works better in combination with other alternative treatments.

LAETRILE (AMYGDALIN, VITAMIN B$_{17}$)

Laetrile, also known as vitamin B$_{17}$, is a treatment that uses amygdalin, a cyanide-containing substance found in many plants, especially almonds, fruit seeds, millet, and buckwheat. The major commercial sources of laetrile are almond and apricot kernels.

Laetrile is believed to kill cancer cells by breaking down into its component molecules of glucose, hydrogen cyanide, and benzaldehyde. Benzaldehyde reacts with cyanide to produce a poison that kills the cancer cells. Laetrile is apparently effective for all types of cancers, and is known best for preventing metastases. It can also reduce pain and has been reported to increase survival time.

Since some laetrile molecules react chemically with an enzyme in non-cancerous cells, rendering them useless for killing cancer cells, you need to take high doses of laetrile over a prolonged period of time—long enough to enable the laetrile molecules to find all the cancer cells. You must also follow a strict diet that builds up trypsin and chymotrypsin, digestive enzymes that break down enzymes surrounding the cancer cell so that white blood cells can kill it.

Laetrile is extremely controversial in the U.S. and is not approved for use here by the FDA. Research done at the Mayo Clinic in the late 1970s concluded that laetrile was not an effective cancer treatment. Advocates for laetrile objected that the study was flawed, using poor-quality laetrile and testing it on patients who had already had conventional chemotherapy. However, conventional medical experts continue to claim that laetrile is both ineffective and toxic.

In fact, laetrile is quite safe, but it's important to take it according to the correct protocol. For greatest effectiveness, laetrile should be taken with vitamin A and pancreatic enzymes. It can be taken in the form of apricot kernels (there is a small soft kernel inside the hard shell). Outside the U.S., you can buy laetrile pills, which must be taken with water on an empty stomach. Do not eat or drink anything for an hour after taking a dose. It is also possible to order injectable laetrile online; this form is better for high doses. Laetrile can be used in conjunction with other alternative therapies.

ISCADOR

Iscador is a fermented water extract of the mistletoe plant, a parasite that grows on trees. Extracts from different trees are used for different types of cancers. Mistletoe has a range of benefits.

- It stimulates the immune system by increasing natural killer cells (an important type of lymphocyte that contains granules with enzymes that can kill tumor cells) and enhancing their activity (the immune connection).

- It decreases the toxicity of cancer cells and inhibits their growth.

- It protects DNA.

- As a bonus, it improves mood and outlook by increasing appetite and energy and reducing pain.

Over 100 studies have investigated the use of mistletoe extract to treat different types of cancer. The only studies on humans, however, were done on breast cancer patients. Compared to the control groups, women receiving mistletoe therapy showed significantly fewer side effects from chemotherapy, and their lives were extended significantly.

Mistletoe is generally used together with conventional treatments to enhance their effectiveness. It is injected under the skin. Some patients do this themselves. But since Iscador is accepted by the FDA as a homeopathic medicine, there are some American doctors who administer it.

UKRAIN

Developed in 1978, Ukrain is a compound created by combining alkaloids from the celandine plant with the chemo drug thiotepa. It's essentially a semi-natural chemotherapy that has no side effects. In experiments on living cells, Ukrain was highly toxic to cancer cells, preventing cancer growth, yet nontoxic to normal cells.[4] Ukrain inhibits angiogenesis (formation of new blood vessels), starving tumors and preventing metastases.

In cancer patients, Ukrain has stimulated the immune system (the immune connection) and caused complete or partial regression of tumors and metastases without harming normal cells, although sometimes the result is simply a long-term stabilization of the cancer. It is administered intravenously or by intramuscular injection. The dose depends on the patient's immune status and the extent of the cancer, as determined by the physician.

Based on the results of two small studies, Ukrain was approved for treatment of pancreatic cancer in the U.S. and Australia. It has also been approved by other countries and is available in Europe and Mexico.

ESCOZINE

Escozine is made from the serum (or venom) of the Caribbean blue scorpion. Initially developed in Cuba starting in 1980, it has been shown to shrink tumors, relieve pain, reduce inflammation (the inflammation connection), and increase survival. Researchers believe that Escozine most likely works by stimulating the body's ability to fight cancer (the immune connection). It combines well with conventional treatments. Clinical studies on humans have shown that Escozine is completely safe, although it occasionally produces brief side effects that can be annoying, such as temporary discomfort in the area where tumors are located.

Escozine is taken orally, although for some types of cancer it is also given in other ways, including by aerosol mist, douche, eyedrops, suppository, or topically. It is not approved by the FDA, but the manufacturer plans to apply to conduct clinical trials in the U.S.

SODIUM BICARBONATE

Sodium bicarbonate (plain old baking soda) is the treatment developed by Dr. Simoncini that I referred to earlier in describing Barbara's case. Dr. Simoncini espouses a theory that cancer is caused by a fungus, and he developed this treatment to kill the fungus. As you no doubt realize, I am not an adherent of this theory; I've already described what I believe causes cancer and my theory of the cancer connections. However I do believe that sodium bicarbonate can sometimes be a useful treatment, because it raises the pH of cancer cells—that is, it addresses the pH connection.

As I explained in the Prologue, cancer cells thrive in an acidic environment. Administering sodium bicarbonate makes cancer cells alkaline and reduces tumor growth. In studies on mice at the Arizona Cancer Center, sodium bicarbonate raised the pH of tumor cells and prevented metastases.[5] Sodium bicarbonate can be given intravenously or taken orally simply by dissolving the correct amount in water. This treatment should be used only under a doctor's supervision.

Many physicians use sodium bicarbonate. In my opinion, however, it is not the most effective treatment. Contrary to what you may hear from conventional physicians, the concept that the body can be made alkaline is certainly valid, and there are therapies that can raise the pH. But oral sodium bicarbonate requires such large doses that patients feel bloated and uncomfortable. Their appetite decreases, compromising their nutritional status, which has already been compromised by the cancer. Another problem with sodium bicarbonate is that it's practically impossible to raise the body's pH higher than 8 (as Simoncini tried to do) because the body naturally strives to remain acidic in order to absorb calcium from food.

What's more, sodium bicarbonate does not actually kill cancer cells. Its only benefit is to slow the aggressiveness of small tumors. So instead of IV sodium bicarbonate, I prefer to use a treatment developed by Dr. Mark Rosenberg, which will be described in Chapter 7.

HYPERTHERMIA

Hyperthermia is the use of heat to treat cancer. Exposing the whole body, or part of the body, to a high temperature damages or kills cancer cells, or makes them more susceptible to conventional radiation and chemotherapy. Because cancer cells cannot tolerate heat as well as normal cells, they start to suffer damage at temperatures over 41°C (106°F). Acidic cells and those in the S (DNA synthesis) phase of the cell cycle are particularly vulnerable.

- In *local hyperthermia,* heat is applied to the area of the tumor, using various devices, depending on whether the tumor is near the surface of the skin, in or near a body cavity, or deep inside the body. The devices emit microwave, ultrasound, or radiofrequency energy.

- In *regional hyperthermia,* a large area such as an entire organ or limb is treated. Different techniques are used depending on the tumor location. For example, to treat liver or lung cancer, doctors remove some of the patient's blood, heat it, and circulate it back into the body, often while administering chemo drugs. Although local and regional hyperthermia are used in many clinics around the world, whole-body hyperthermia is much more popular.

- In *whole-body or systemic hyperthermia,* the entire body is heated to an internal temperature of 41–42°C (106–108°F) for about two hours, or to 39–40°C (102–104°F) for four to eight hours. The goal is to reproduce the curative effects of fever which, as physicians have known since ancient times, has a therapeutic effect in all sorts of disorders. During the treatment, the patient lies in a special chamber that encloses the entire body except for the head. Most hyperthermia units use infrared radiation. The temperature is steadily increased, maintained for a predetermined time (thirty minutes to several hours), then slowly cooled. The patient is usually sedated and asleep during the entire procedure.

Hyperthermia for many types of cancer has been well studied, though most of these studies involved advanced-stage disease, where the treatment was a last resort. Hyperthermia induced remission in some patients and partial remission in others, and relieved pain and other symptoms, such as loss of appetite.

Hyperthermia increases the immune response, for example by making natural killer cells more vigilant in finding and attacking cancer cells. It stimulates the dendritic cells that are used in cancer vaccines (*see* chapter 5). It makes chemotherapy and radiation more effective, and it works well in conjunction with other alternative treatments, including IPT, vitamin C, and oxidative therapies. Whole-body hyperthermia causes a series of reactions in cancer cells that makes them unable to generate energy and leads to a buildup of lactic acid inside the cells as well as the production of special proteins called heat-shock proteins, which cause cell apoptosis—a great setup for cancer destruction. So you see that hyperthermia addresses three cancer connections: the oxygen, pH, and immune connections.

Hyperthermia is used frequently in Europe and elsewhere in the world as an adjuvant therapy, part of an integrative approach. In the U.S., however, it is still considered experimental and is available at only a few clinics.

DMSO

Dimethyl sulfoxide, or DMSO, is a natural solvent, a by-product of the wood industry. It easily penetrates the skin and other tissues, and can carry other drugs along with it. Used in combination with chemo drugs, it targets cancer cells, delivering the drugs to these cells more efficiently, so lower doses of chemotherapy can be used. Many integrative doctors use DMSO in conjunction with another treatment, insulin potentiation therapy (IPT, *see* Chapter 4). A study done on rats concluded that DMSO delayed the spread of cancer and prolonged survival rates.

DMSO is FDA approved only for treatment of interstitial cystitis (bladder inflammation), but doctors can prescribe it legally off-label for treating cancer. Its anti-inflammatory action can restore normal function in damaged cells, addressing the inflammation connection. DMSO also has antioxidant properties and may interfere with cancer growth.

DMSO is administered intravenously on its own or during IPT treatment.

THYMUS

Thymosin alpha 1 is a substance produced by the thymus gland. Zadaxin is a synthetic version of thymosin, called thymalfasin, that stimulates the immune system by triggering production of natural killer cells, T cells, and T-helper cells (thus addressing the immune connection). Zadaxin also slows the breakdown of T cells and increases production of inter-feron gamma and interleukin-2, substances that are part of the immune response. Zadaxin has recently been approved by the FDA as an orphan drug (a drug being developed to treat rare diseases) for treatment of malignant melanoma.

Zadaxin is generally given twice a week by subcutaneous injection. It is approved in thirty countries as a cancer adjuvant therapy and is used in conjunction with other alternative treatments (hydrogen peroxide, IPT, ozone, and vitamin C).

SALICINIUM

Salicinium is a natural plant-derived substance that has several anti-cancer effects. First, it interferes with the process of fermentation. Salicinium is a complex sugar, and an enzyme called 6-glucosidase is needed to break it down. Normal cells don't have this enzyme, so they don't break down salicinium, which has no effect on them. But cancer cells do have 6-glucosidase, which they use to break down salicinium. Just like vitamin

C, salicinium fools the cancer cells into thinking it's sugar, without actually providing the nutrition they need.

Salicinium also blocks mitosis (cell division) of cancer cells and makes fermenting cancer cells susceptible to attack by the immune system by blocking nagalase, an enzyme these cancer cells need to protect themselves from the immune system. Blocking nagalase enables macrophages to confidently perform their noble function of recognizing and destroying cancer cells. Salicinium thus addresses the genetic, immune, and sugar connections.

A study of 250 Stage IV breast cancer patients treated with salicinium showed an overall response rate of 79 percent at thirty-three months, with no significant side effects.

Salicinium is a great adjunct to both conventional chemo and IPT. It is first given intravenously over a period of three weeks, then taken orally in a form called Orasal. Salicinium must be used with pHenomenal, a supplement that removes excess hydrogen molecules from the body, making it more alkaline, and thus addressing the pH connection.

CARNIVORA

Carnivora is an extract of the Venus flytrap plant. In 1988, plumbagin, the active component of Carnivora, was isolated and proved to be a powerful immune stimulant. Since that time about 2,000 people, including the late President Ronald Reagan, have been treated with Carnivora. Carnivora is used mainly to treat immune disorders, particularly HIV infection and cancer, with varying degrees of success. Studies have shown that this product can reduce tumor weight and size, without any side effects.

Carnivora is taken orally in the form of drops, again in combination with other treatments. So here is one more therapy that addresses the immune connection.

FINAL THOUGHTS

I hope that reading this chapter has helped to convince you that alternative/integrative therapies can indeed help fight cancer. And perhaps you don't care very much that some experts describe these treatments as unproven, unscientific, and experimental because you are now aware that their proof lies in their success—in the experiences of thousands of cancer survivors whom they have helped considerably. Above all, it's important to keep your eye on several facts.

- These therapies work;

- They have no side effects; and

- They're less expensive than their conventional counterparts.

In describing conventional cancer treatment, I use the phrase *the conventional trio.* But in talking about alternative treatments, it makes more sense to talk about an integrative/alternative *orchestra,* considering their great range and variety of roles. Who plays what role in this orchestra's performance? Obviously, the physician is the conductor. He or she writes the musical arrangements, chooses the instruments, and decides which musicians will play.

So, among this ensemble, who plays lead violin? Very often this role is played by insulin potentiation therapy, which the next chapter will discuss in great detail. The therapies described in this chapter—and those described in chapters 5 through 8—play all the other instruments. One more important consideration: in order for this orchestra to be in perfect harmony, every instrument must play impeccably. Otherwise no one will enjoy the symphony.

CHAPTER 4

- - - - -

Insulin Potentiation Therapy—
Tough Insulin, Gentle Chemo

INITIAL THOUGHTS

If you just read the long list of possible alternative cancer treatments in Chapter 3, your head is probably spinning with questions. Which treatment is the most important? The most powerful? And which one is your physician most likely to choose for your particular type of cancer?

Certainly it's impossible to use the entire alternative kitchen sink of treatments at the same time. So when integrative physicians encounter a new patient, they ask, "What therapy should I use to begin an aggressive treatment program for this person?" This question goes through my mind every time I treat someone with advanced metastatic cancer. Most often, I answer it by starting the person's regimen with the very special treatment known as insulin potentiation therapy (IPT).

IPT isn't the only treatment I use in my anti-cancer program. It must be given in conjunction with intravenous vitamin C, as well as some of the other treatments described in this book. But it's definitely the treatment I rely on most. IPT has a smart-bomb ability to target cancer cells, causing them major damage and possibly destroying them completely. In IPT, insulin is administered to make cancer-cell membranes more permeable so chemo drugs can get inside the cells more easily. Because of the insulin, far lower doses of chemo drugs are needed, which means you experience few, if any, side effects. At the same time, normal cells are not harmed. IPT helps people feel better, live longer, and, as many integrative physicians and their patients will tell you, enjoy a much better quality of life.

It's no surprise, then, that the founders of the Best Answer for Cancer Foundation—both of whom licked their own cancer with IPT—describe the IPT experience as "thriving while surviving."

THE BEST ANSWER FOR CANCER FOUNDATION

This organization was founded by Annie Brandt and Rachel Best in 2004. It consists of doctors and patients working to shift the cancer paradigm from a one-size-fits-all, disease-based approach to a patient-centered, integrative medical approach. The foundation's goal is to bring education and research to people around the world and to assist them in making difficult decisions as they choose their treatment options for surviving. At its website (www.bestanswerforcancer.org) you can find more information on alternative treatments and join the online forum where you can ask questions and share experiences and information with patients, survivors, caregivers, and other concerned people.

I am a proud member of this foundation, so I gladly accepted an invitation to attend their Ninth Annual International IPT/IPT-LD Conference in 2011, but quite honestly, without great expectations. (In 2006 the term IPT was changed to IPT-LD—Insulin Potentiation Targeted Low-Dose Chemotherapy—in an attempt to better describe it. However, IPT and IPT-LD are the same thing.) I anticipated a small gathering of people sharing experiences and exchanging ideas. But what I found was 160 attendees who brought a level of energy and enthusiasm comparable to that produced by the three to six thousand attendees you would find at a conventional medicine cancer conference. All the speakers were exciting, they offered extremely useful information and innovative views. IPT-LD was the cornerstone of the conference. Throughout this book I'll be offering you leading-edge information from this event.

Foundation co-founders Rachel Best and Annie Brandt met each other as IPT patients. Rachel Best had had a course of conventional chemo for ovarian cancer. Her cancer recurred in 2004, but responded well to IPT treatments. Sadly, however, she died in 2006 due to an infection she caught in the hospital after routine surgery that was not related to her cancer.

The story of Annie Brandt, Rachel Best's co-founder, provides an example and a challenge for every person with cancer. She is living proof that an integrative approach really works, and for that she deserves a special place in this book.

THE ANNIE BRANDT STORY

Annie Brandt's story began in 1992, with a diagnosis of chronic fatigue and immune dysfunction syndrome (CFIDS), a condition for which no conventional treatment existed. Forced to explore non-conventional therapies, including diet, vitamins and herbs, mind/body medicine, and spirituality, she discovered an entire world of healing knowledge outside conventional medicine. She developed her own program and used it to heal her immune system and her subsequent health problems that included multiple sclerosis, a heart problem, and chemical sensitivities. After a lengthy round of therapies, she thought she had restored her health.

Then, in July 2001, she found a lump under her arm that was diagnosed as breast cancer, at least stage II, and probably more advanced (the doctors could not say for sure since the tumor could not be seen on imaging tests). Her surgeon advised a double mastectomy followed by chemo and radiation and offered to fit Annie in on the following Tuesday. Brandt went home in a state of shock, prepared to follow this advice. But after a friend's prodding, she snapped out of it and dropped what she calls "the sheep method"—blindly doing what she was told. Over the weekend, she did extensive research and concluded that, given her precarious health, submitting to the conventional trio of treatments, with the stress and side effects they entailed, would further weaken her delicate immune system, make the cancer stronger, and ultimately kill her. On Monday she told her doctor that she would not have the surgery, but would instead search out alternative methods. The doctor responded that there was little hope for her.

Brandt recalls, "I had the double-edged benefit of *knowing without a doubt* that that conventional cancer therapy would kill me fairly quickly and unpleasantly. The good news, to me, was that I would not have to try to fight the cancer while dealing with all of the side effects of conventional therapy. The bad news was that, whatever I chose to do, I would be doing it against the mainstream of medical experience and knowledge."[1]

Further scans revealed cancer in Brandt's lungs and brain, so her doctors changed the diagnosis to advanced stage 4 metastatic breast cancer. (True to her nature, however, she refused to allow them to specify the stage, believing this would have an adverse effect on her entire mind/body system.) Brandt says the oncologist suggested that "I get my affairs in order."

Now she had to face the reactions of her friends and family, who put intense pressure on her to change her mind. She explained what she had learned through her research and why conventional treatment was not an option for her. "Eventually," Brandt says, "they left me alone and waited for me to die."

Instead, she went back to her research. She learned that most cancer survivors had not used one single treatment, but had followed a coordinated program. She tweaked the modalities she had already used to overcome her immune-system dysfunction, and added detoxification, lifestyle changes, and immune system boosters to her own regimen. She stayed on it for a year—longer than the doctors had expected her to live—until she discovered new, enlarged lymph nodes. "I knew the cancer was on the move again and that I needed to add a formal cancer therapy to my holistic platform . . . I knew I had to add something very powerful."

At this point, Brandt discovered IPT/IPT-LD and was amazed to learn that, though it had been successfully used for cancer since 1946, hardly anyone knew about it, and conventional oncologists did not provide it. Brandt, who lived in southern Texas, chose to go to Mexico to be treated by Dr. Donato Perez Garcia III, the grandson of the physician who invented IPT. The treatment took only an hour, and afterward Annie went out to shop and have some fun.

"Yes," she says, "I had fun during that treatment, and every other treatment after that . . . My research had shown me that laughter and fun would boost the immune system and light up the frontal lobe of the brain, effectively canceling out fear and proving to be anti-cancer."

The treatments caused no side effects; she had lots of energy, and she continued to lead her regular life.

Then in December 2002, the tumor became visible by ultrasound, since IPT had reduced the inflammation in the breast tissue. Once more

Brandt's oncologist recommended mastectomy, once more she refused, and by March 2003, her tests showed no indication of cancer. Typically, the oncologist steadfastly resisted the idea that IPT had healed Brandt's cancer, choosing to believe instead that her case was one of spontaneous remission.

July 4, 2012 was the anniversary of Annie Brandt's diagnosis, marking the eleventh year of her survival.

THE IPT STORY—HOW IT ALL STARTED

IPT began with the Mexican physician Donato Perez Garcia I, M.D. (1891–1971). In 1930, learning of the just-discovered hormone insulin, he used it to successfully self-treat a gastrointestinal disorder he had. Believing the insulin helped his body assimilate food better, he theorized it might also improve the assimilation of medicines. He went on to treat various diseases by first administering insulin in order to cause a state of low blood sugar (hypoglycemia), then administering whatever drug was indicated for the condition he was treating. His first patient was Carlos Sosa, who had neurosyphilis (syphilis of the brain, at that time considered incurable). Dr. Perez Garcia gave Sosa low doses of insulin together with a combination of mercury and arsenic, then the standard treatment for syphilis. Sosa recovered and survived another forty years. For him, Dr. Perez Garcia's treatment was a gift of life.

In 1943, Dr. Perez Garcia was invited to the San Diego Naval Hospital, where he very successfully treated patients with neurosyphilis, cholecystitis, rheumatic fever, and malaria. A 1944 issue of *Time* described his work as "Insulin for Everything."

IPT was first used for the treatment of cancer in 1947, when the first chemotherapy drugs became available. One person with squamous cell carcinoma of the tongue received fractionated (small) doses of conventional chemo combined with the IPT treatments and lived disease-free for another thirty years.

THE UNCONVENTIONAL TRIO OF IPT/IPT-LD

Now I want to introduce to you two more Mexican physicians and an American one: Dr. Donato Perez Garcia II, son of Perez Garcia I; his son,

Dr. Donato Perez Garcia III; and Steven G. Ayre, M.D., a pioneer of IPT in the U.S. In summer 1976 Dr. Ayre received training in IPT from Dr. Perez Garcia II, who had followed in his father's path. Then Drs. Ayre and Perez Garcia II worked closely together to develop IPT. Their research and clinical trials led to publication of five articles in peer-reviewed journals and a number of scientific presentations.

In 1996, they reported their findings at the 42d Annual Symposium on Fundamental Cancer Research at the MD Anderson Institute in Houston. Following this event, MD Anderson established its own Center for Alternative Medicine Research. An Anderson investigator visited Dr. Perez Garcia II's clinic in Mexico City and that of Dr. Perez Garcia III in Tijuana. He left completely convinced of the value of IPT and exclaimed, "This is incredible. How come nothing has ever been done about this before?"

In 1997, the unconventional trio presented their findings at the National Institutes of Health (NIH) Office of Alternative Medicine POMES (Practice Outcome Monitoring Evaluation System) Conference. In 2000, Drs. Perez Garcia II and Ayre made a Best Case Series presentation before the Cancer Advisory Panel of the NIH Office of Complementary and Alternative Medicine. They were asked to develop more data and make another such presentation in the future.

Today over forty board-certified IPT practitioners perform IPT treatments in their offices and clinics around the world. And I am one of them. As a student of Dr. Ayre, who trained me, I'm proud to be an offspring of the father of American IPT—one of the greatest IPT physicians in the world.

WHAT EXACTLY IS IPT?

IPT-LD is actually a specific use of FDA-approved drugs, consisting of off-label insulin and chemotherapy agents. The role played by the chemo drugs is obvious: they kill cancer cells. Insulin takes advantage of this powerful ability of chemo drugs but enables them to be used in much lower doses, avoiding almost all the side effects of chemotherapy. In conventional chemotherapy, most of the drugs administered aren't taken up by the cancer cells. Doctors use large doses so the cancer cells will absorb enough drugs to kill them. The rest of the drug dose damages healthy cells. IPT, by contrast, uses insulin to open the cancer cell walls so that far more of the drugs get into the cells. As a result, IPT requires only about one-tenth of the standard doses.

When most people hear about IPT, they have two questions:

1. What in the world does insulin have to do with chemo?

2. What use is a low dose of chemo drugs? It's not really enough to kill cancer cells, is it?

Not enough research has been done to specify the exact mechanism by which IPT works, but let me explain the theory that's been developed so far. The two keys to IPT's effectiveness are insulin and insulin-like growth factor (IGF). As you know, insulin is the powerful hormone used to treat diabetes. Secreted by the pancreas in healthy people, insulin has many physiological functions, but the main one is to deliver glucose across cell membranes into the cells. You could say that insulin creates a communications link across the cell membrane by opening specific insulin receptors located on the outer surface of the membrane. It is through this opening that the chemo drugs get into the cell.

In the Prologue, I explained that cancer cells require large amounts of glucose to generate energy. They secrete their own insulin in order to absorb all this glucose. Cancer-cell membranes contain many more insulin receptors than normal cells. In the presence of insulin, these receptors open channels in the cell membrane so they can take in more glucose—and it is at this point that the chemo drugs are administered, and can then enter the cells as easily as glucose.

Insulin has a second benefit as well. Cancer cells can stimulate their own division and growth by secreting IGF, and they have many more IGF receptors than normal cells. At any given time, not all cancer cells are in the cell-division phase; they usually take turns dividing. But insulin affects the IGF receptors by triggering rapid division of non-dividing cells. Thus when the chemo drugs hit the cancer cells, a much larger proportion are in the S (growing) phase of the cell cycle, when they are most vulnerable. Using insulin to increase the number of cells in the S phase produces a dramatic increase in the tumor-killing effect of chemo drugs.

WHAT THE RESEARCH SAYS

Laboratory studies have reported that insulin increases the cell-killing effect of the chemo drug methotrexate up to 10,000 times. Other laboratory studies have shown that adding insulin to breast cancer cells causes a 66 percent increase in the number of cells undergoing the S phase of the cell cycle, in comparison to only 37 percent in control groups to which insulin was not added.

In 2003, a study was conducted with thirty women who had metastatic breast cancer that was resistant to a combination of fluorouracil, Adriamycin, and cyclophosphamide, as well as to hormone therapy. The study's purpose was to investigate insulin's clinical value as a facilitator of methotrexate. Three groups of ten women each received two twenty-one-day courses of treatment. One group got insulin plus methotrexate, another got methotrexate by itself, and the third got insulin by itself. Each patient's target tumor was measured before and after treatment. The investigators found that the increase in the size of the tumor was significantly lower among the women who received insulin together with methotrexate than among the other two groups. They concluded that the insulin had enhanced the anti-cancer effect of the methotrexate.[2]

So it is clear that IPT insulin acts not just as a facilitator, but also as a biological response modifier. That is, it modifies the biological response of the cancer-cell membranes to allow more anti-cancer drugs into the cells, making the drugs much more effective. And it modifies the growth characteristics of the tumor, making it more susceptible to the drugs. What a brilliant example of synergistic work by two potent pharmaceutical agents—insulin and chemo.

How does this gate-opening effect actually work? According to Steven Ayre, insulin activates an enzyme known as delta-9 desaturase. This enzyme causes the breakdown of stearic acid—a component of the cell wall with a melting point of 68°C—into oleic acid, which has a much lower melting point of 5°C. At the normal body temperature of 36°C, the cell membrane becomes very fluid and much more permeable—and that's what opens the gate to the chemo drugs.

IPT AND THE CANCER CONNECTIONS

By lowering blood-sugar levels, IPT-LD addresses both the sugar connection and the MID connection. Lowering blood-sugar levels normalizes elevated cholesterol and triglyceride blood levels. In turn, the level of cholesterol in lymphocytes drops, helping reverse the condition of immunodepression. You see, then, how powerful and effective the IPT smart-bomb really is.

WHAT'S AN IPT TREATMENT LIKE?

Most IPT treatments take place in the physician's office, and begin with placement of a standard IV drip of saline solution into a vein in the arm. This drip keeps the vein open, making it easy to administer the insulin, chemo drugs, other medications, and, at the end of the treatment, a glucose solution to restore the normal blood-sugar level.

After all the drugs to be used are prepared, the insulin is administered through the IV line, and every ten minutes the patient's sugar level is tested by finger sticks until the desired level of 45–40 mg/ml is reached. At this point, the patient usually complains of feeling hot, sweaty, and sometimes mildly confused. This is known as the *therapeutic moment*— the right moment to administer the chemo medications through the IV.

Once all these drugs have been given, a glucose solution is given to bring the glucose level back to normal. The patient also gets Gatorade to replenish sugar and potassium and can, at this point, enjoy a meal (which she/he has been told to bring along). Generally, the sugar level goes up within ten minutes, and the patient feels less hot and more clear-headed. When the sugar level is at 100–120 mg/ml, the treatment is complete. Usually the entire procedure takes ninety minutes, though the exact timing of the treatment depends on the nature of the disease, the person's condition, and how quickly the blood-sugar level drops in response to the insulin.

Unlike conventional chemo, which is given only every few weeks, it is possible to give IPT treatments twice a week at the beginning, (sometimes three times a week), then once a week. The advantage of more frequent treatments is that the cancer cells don't have time to recuperate between treatments. To avoid development of resistance to the chemo drugs, the drug combination administered is routinely altered.

NO—IPT-LD IS NOT DANGEROUS

The naysaying physicians claim that IPT presents various hazards due to complications of hypoglycemia—particularly a risk of hypoglycemic coma, should the blood sugar drop to a dangerously low level. I can assure you that hypoglycemia is very easily controlled by IV administration of a glucose solution. As many people with diabetes know, when symptoms of hypoglycemia develop, two pieces of candy or a glass of orange juice will quickly take care of them. It's a condition that's very easy to reverse. And please note: there has been not a single case of mortality from IPT.

In case you're wondering whether people with diabetes can have IPT, the answer is definitely yes. The only difference is that it takes somewhat longer to bring their elevated sugar levels down to achieve the therapeutic moment.

Choosing Chemo Drugs for IPT—Special Tests

As everyone has been told, medicine is an art, not a science. And choosing the combination of chemotherapy drugs for a particular patient really is a work of art, since getting the combination right may determine the treatment's success or failure. In part, integrative physicians use exactly the same approach as conventional oncologists to determine the best combination: they take into consideration the type of tumor, the results of lab tests of biopsied cancer cells (which reveal tumor type and some specific characteristics, such as estrogen sensitivity in breast cancer), the reported results of the efficacy of different drugs in large clinical studies, and the physician's own previous experience.

But IPT practitioners also make much greater use than conventional oncologists of so-called chemosensitivity tests, which personalize the treatment by determining the sensitivity of an individual's tumor to specific drugs. Some of these tests use tissue analysis; the cancer cells are tested in special labs against different chemo drugs, in the same way that conventional medicine determines the sensitivities of different microbes to antibiotics by culturing cells from urine, blood, or sputum. Other chemosensitivity tests use blood samples to examine circulating tumor cells (CTC) for sensitivity.

Another, important type of chemosensitivity test is based on genetic analysis of cancer cells. Such tests use molecular biology techniques to detect the specific genes necessary for the cancer's growth and survival, thereby enabling the physician to choose drugs that target these genes. Such specific, individualized testing is extremely valuable for making the best use of expensive and toxic chemo drugs. Most types of tumors can be tested—breast, cervical, colon, gastrointestinal, hematological, kidney, leukemia, liver, lung, lymphoma, ovarian, prostate, skin, and many others.

Another advantage of genetic-based testing has to do with the fact that a number of chemo drugs—among them cyclophosphamide and irinontecan—are virtually inactive in their original form and need to be activated once they enter the body, for example by liver enzymes. This requirement means that they cannot be tested in the lab for chemosensitivity. A conventional doctor's choice to use one of these drugs is like shooting an arrow into the sky—he doesn't know if it'll work or not. But a chemosensitivity test that uses genetic profiling does not depend on prior activization of the drug being tested, so the physician can aim the arrow right at the bull's-eye.

One chemosensitivity test, known as the *Greek test,* is conducted by Research Genetic Cancer Centre (RGCC), a lab in Greece. Isolated malignant cells that the physician obtains by a patented technique are tested not only against various chemo drugs, but also against biological-response modifiers—agents such as ascorbic acid, CoQ_{10}, hydrogen peroxide, mistletoe, and Ukrain, that boost the immune system, relieve side effects, and may also have an anti-cancer effect. Another test, conducted by Biofocus, a German lab, provides essentially the same information. Similar labs are opening elsewhere. As gene-based chemosensitivity testing enters more widespread use, the technique will be further improved.

Since conventional oncologists rarely use tissue tests to determine which drugs to prescribe, such testing is done by patient request, in most cases. Unfortunately, few patients are aware that these tests even exist and can't take advantage of them. In order to have such a test, you must ask the surgeon to preserve tissue for it from the biopsy.

JILL'S AMAZING STORY

One case presented at the International IPT/IPT-LD Conference, describing a woman treated with IPT, is so extraordinary that I want to share it with you.

In December 2010, a fifty-five-year-old woman named Jill came to see Dr. Juergen Winkler, an integrative physician in Oceanside, CA. She complained of abdominal pain that had begun four months earlier, along with poor appetite, weight loss, and severe fatigue. This was the first time she had consulted a doctor for these problems, and she came only because her boyfriend, who was extremely concerned about her health, had more or less dragged her there.

Dr. Winkler's physical exam revealed a mass in Jill's left breast, enlarged lymph nodes in her left armpit, and a hugely enlarged, tender liver with multiple nodules. He suspected metastatic left breast cancer and did an abdominal ultrasound, which showed many lesions that involved 80 percent of Jill's liver.

The results of a blood test made it clear that Jill's condition was extremely serious. Her liver function was highly abnormal. To take just one result, her ammonia level was over 250 (the normal range is 15–45). The most troubling sign was that her CA 27.29 tumor marker (which indicates breast-cancer metastasis) was 12,264. The normal range is 0–38.5.

Dr. Winkler immediately sent Jill for a PET/CT scan and a biopsy. He also sent a blood sample to the Research Genetic Cancer Centre (RGCC) for a chemosensitivity test. A week later, the initial results showed widespread bone metastasis, severe liver metastasis involving 80 percent of the liver, and left breast cancer, with swollen lymph nodes in the armpit, right lung, and the rear part of the abdomen. The core needle liver biopsy revealed breast adenocarcinoma of both breasts that had metastasized.

You may wonder how all of this could develop without Jill ever coming to a doctor. Like many people, she feared she had cancer, but was more afraid of the chemotherapy than of the cancer itself. The only reason she agreed to consult Dr. Winkler was that she knew he practiced integrative medicine.

Since the case was clearly so serious, even before the biopsy and other test results came in, Dr. Winkler administered an IPT treatment using Taxol, Adriamycin, and methotrexate—the most common drug combination for breast cancer. At the therapeutic moment, he also administered DMSO along with the chemo drugs. Once Jill's sugar level had returned to normal after the IPT, she also received a high dose of vitamin C and a solution of free amino acids through the IV line. The free amino acids (free meaning not chemically combined with another substance) provided protein to improve her nutritional status.

The next week, Jill had two more of the same IPT treatments. At this point, she noticed she had less pain and her energy level had increased. Results now came in from RGCC, showing that her cancer was sensitive to six specific chemo drugs. One of these, carboplatin, was added to the fourth IPT treatment. For the fifth treatment, Jill was given a different combination from among the six drugs; the idea was to avoid chemoresistance by alternating drugs. After her twelfth treatment, and after receiving several different drug combinations, Jill's CA 27.29 tumor marker had dropped to 930, while her ammonia level was down to 60, indicating improvement in her liver function.

Dr. Winkler now put Jill on a regimen of Arimidex once a day, ultraviolet radiation of blood (see Chapter 6), injections of Iscador, and oral low-dose naltrexone (LDN) for immune stimulation. (Naltrexone is a drug approved by the FDA for use in helping overcome drug and alcohol addiction; it's used off-label to boost the immune system. See Chapter 7.) In March 2011, Jill's PET/CT report came back with this comment from the radiologist: "Dramatic response to interval treatment [i.e., treatment since the last PET scan]." Both breast masses were smaller, and the PET scan revealed reduced abdominal lymph nodes and a reduction of 70 percent in the size of her liver.

During this entire period, Jill's only side effects were a very minor loss of hair and one episode of low white-cell blood count that was rectified by an injection of Neupogen (filgrastim, a drug that stimulates the bone marrow to produce white blood cells).

A large number of favorable responses to IPT have been reported by physicians around the globe. Jill's case provides one more powerful example of how effective this treatment can be.

In my own experience, as well as that of many other integrative physicians, chemosensitivity blood tests are a great help in 30 to 40 percent of cases. Tissue tests are far more helpful. I expect, though, that the blood tests will become more sophisticated, providing better guidance in choosing drugs, and will be used more widely in the future.

The effectiveness of the IPT chemo combinations is generally monitored by regularly checking the tumor markers and doing PET/CT and MRI scans. For breast, colon, and prostate tumors, there's a brand-new test called CellSearch developed by Johnson & Johnson, which detects circulating tumor cells in the blood. The normal value of this test is 0. Any higher number indicates that the tumor is progressing, and the chemo combination needs to be changed. The advantage of CellSearch is that it can be done every month, since it only requires drawing blood— there's no radiation or discomfort—which means it is possible to monitor patients much more closely and easily.

IPT AND THE GENETIC CONNECTION

I've discussed how IPT's use of insulin addresses the sugar and MID cancer connections. IPT's use of chemo drugs also addresses the genetic connection, since the way these drugs kill tumor cells is by attacking their genetic material, DNA and RNA. Here is how some of these brave destroyers work.

The chemo drugs 6-mercaptopurine, 6-thioguanine, and methotrexate inhibit synthesis of purines, proteins arranged in a ring shape that cells use to make the building blocks of DNA and RNA. Cytarabine, by contrast, inhibits DNA synthesis directly. The group of chemo drugs called alkylating agents (among them cytoxan, leukeran, temodar, carboplatin, thiotepa) prevent cell division by creating abnormal links between the strands of DNA. When the DNA is thus altered, the cell cannot divide and multiply. Antimetabolites, another group of drugs (methotrexate, fluorouracil, 6-mercaptopurine, and others), have structures similar to those of the naturally occurring compounds that cells use to synthesize DNA and RNA. The drugs take the place of these natural compounds, preventing the cell from dividing—just like vitamin C fooling the cancer cell into thinking that it's sugar.

TYPES OF CANCER TREATABLE BY IPT

Adenocarcinoma of unknown primary origin

Astrocytoma

Biliary

Bladder

Breast

Carcinoid tumor

Carcinomas

Cervical

Chondrosarcoma

Colon

Differentiated carcinomas

Endometrial

Epidermoid carcinoma

Esophageal

Ewing's sarcoma (pediatric)

Fibrosarcoma

Gastric

Glioblastoma

Head and neck

Kaposi's sarcoma

Leiomyosarcomas

Leukemia, AML

Leukemia, chronic lymphocytic

Leukemia, chronic myelogenous

Leukemia, hairy cell

Lip

Liver

Lung cancer (non-small-cell)

Lung cancer (small cell)

Lymphoma (pediatric)

Lymphoma, Hodgkin's

Lymphoma, Non-Hodgkin's

Melanoma

Mouth

Mucinous tumors

Multiple myeloma

Mycosis fungoides

Osteosarcoma (pediatric)

Ovarian

Pancreatic

Prostate

Rectal

Renal

Rhabdomyosarcoma

Sarcoma

Sarcomas (bony/soft tissue, pediatric)

Seminomas

Serous tumors

Skin

Small cell carcinoma

Small intestine

Squamous cell carcinoma

Teratomas

Testicular

Throat

Thyroid

Undifferentiated carcinomas

Uterine

Vulva and vaginal

WHAT ARE IPT'S CHANCES OF SUCCESS?

When anyone in the early stages of cancer is treated with IPT right after receiving a diagnosis and having a biopsy, its success rate is about 100 percent. In advanced cases, those who undergo IPT will not necessarily eliminate their cancers completely, but they do all get the benefits I've described. They enjoy an improved quality of life and often live longer, achieving partial and sometimes even complete remission.

IPT can be used as the main therapy for bladder, breast, kidney, ovarian, pancreatic, prostate, and uterine cancer; small cell lung cancer, cancers of the gastrointestinal tract, chronic leukemia, Hodgkin's lymphoma, non-Hodgkin's lymphoma, and sarcomas. It is also useful in treating many other types of cancer. (*See* page 97 for a full list.)

IPT can also be a valuable form of aggressive therapy. In some cases an aggressive cancerous growth creates life-threatening cachexia (muscle wasting), systemic swelling (of the entire body), severe pain, breathing problems, and compression of the spinal cord, conditions for which aggressive treatment is needed. IPT can step up and serve that function. In such cases, IPT spells relief.

FINAL THOUGHTS—
WHY IS IPT NOT A MAINSTREAM TREATMENT?

Many people wonder about this. Why indeed is IPT popular only among alternative and integrative physicians? It uses FDA-approved pharmaceutical drugs, chosen exactly the same as in conventional oncology and used as indicated by all conventional oncology texts. It doesn't produce the side effects that make people feel miserable during standard chemo treatments. It's not merely *as* effective as standard chemo—it's *more* effective. And yet it's less expensive than standard chemo (it uses only a tenth of the standard dose).

One rather flimsy explanation for IPT not being considered a mainstream therapy is that many conventional oncologists don't know it exists. But then you have to ask, why not? IPT has been in use for eighty-one years, more than enough time to learn about and recognize this wonderful life-saving method. So why do only integrative/alternative physicians gladly accept it and use it?

When Annie Brandt asked her oncologist this question, he responded that IPT-LD was considered *experimental* because no clinical trials had been done on it . So she wondered why such a promising treatment *hadn't* been tested. And what she heard from the pharmaceutical companies was what it's always about with big pharma—money. Since the drugs already had FDA approval, the companies were unwilling to bear the expense of further trials—especially because, if IPT did actually become mainstream, they would wind up selling smaller amounts of the drugs.

In my opinion integrative oncologists are "prisoners of truth," to borrow an expression from my good friend Dr. Majid Ali, one of the greatest integrative physicians. He and I know this treatment is not as popular as conventional treatment, but we use it because it *works*. And the truth is that IPT is very well tolerated by all cancer patients. In fact, by contrast with those on standard chemo, who are terrified to step into the treatment room, IPT patients come willingly for their treatments.

- The truth is that IPT has been used successfully to treat cancer for over seventy years in other countries, and about eleven years in the U.S.

- The truth is that the use of insulin in IPT might become just as important as its use in diabetes. That's why some experts describe IPT as *the second discovery of insulin.*

- The truth is that integrative physicians are willing to go beyond the limits of conventional treatment and pursue all possible options that exist now and will exist in the future in order to help their patients survive.

- The truth is that IPT brings remission in those with very difficult-to-treat advanced cancer and sometimes in those with very rare forms of cancer.

- The truth is that IPT can often be used effectively when the person is too weak, or the immune system too depressed, for standard chemo. Or simply when patients flatly refuse standard chemo because they can't take it any longer.

- The truth is that IPT produces very few side effects, mostly occasional constipation, easily manageable mild nausea, and an occasional drop in the white or red blood cell count after the first couple of treatments. That's why many physicians and their patients call it "the kinder, gentler cancer treatment."

- The truth is that not one single case of a fatal complication caused by IPT has ever been reported in its eighty-one years of existence. Someone please tell me what other treatment can make such a claim?

- The truth is that IPT is becoming more popular, and the demand for it is growing. There is no reason why it should not become a standard, conventional treatment for cancer. The only question is when this will happen.

CHAPTER 5

— — — —

Immunotherapy
and Cancer Vaccines

INITIAL THOUGHTS

Many professionals who treat and care for people with cancer—not just oncologists, but scientists, researchers, hospital administrators, and drug and insurance company officials—are frustrated and dissatisfied by the failure of the conventional trio to successfully treat advanced and metastatic cancer. A 2004 article in *Fortune* magazine titled "Why We're Losing the War on Cancer" pointed out that very little research focuses on the mechanisms of metastasis, simply because metastasis is such a difficult phenomenon to investigate.[1] The result is that, despite hundreds of billions of dollars spent on cancer research, there is still no effective conventional therapy for metastatic cancers.

After the death of Massachusetts senator Edward Kennedy from the deadly brain cancer glioblastoma multiforme, the scientific and medical community realized once again how little progress had been made since the war on cancer was declared in 1971. So it's understandable that researchers feel pressure to search for new treatments—new techniques, new medications, new *anything* that might do *something*. In this environment, the latest bandwagon that everyone involved in cancer research has jumped aboard is cancer immunotherapy.

Contemplating this current trend, I sigh with relief. Someone has finally realized that the old concept, *cut it, zap it, kill it,* is generally not useful in advanced cases. Applying these standard therapies to advanced cancer is like trying to knock down a stone wall by giving it a little push with your hand. So I'm glad that researchers have accepted the idea of enlisting the healing forces already within the body and have begun to figure out how to use a person's own immune system as an ally in fighting cancer. And I'm pleased that immunotherapy—a method that has been in wide use by many alternative doctors for several decades—is currently getting a well-deserved boost. Characteristically, however, conventional oncology bases its immunotherapy on expensive drugs that are actually less effective than many alternative therapies—they're just much more extensively promoted.

ADDRESSING THE IMMUNE CONNECTION WITH CANCER IMMUNOTHERAPY

By definition, cancer immunotherapy uses the power of a person's own immune system to attack and destroy tumor cells. As I've explained, however, cancer cells are clever and devious. Many types of cancer cells develop some degree of resistance to their host's immune system.

Simply because tumor cells live inside a person's body, they are in essence that person's own cells. They can carry self-antigens (an antigen is a protein or other type of molecule that triggers a specific immune response) that tell the immune system they are normal cells. What's more, not every attack by immune-system forces destroys its target. Cancer cells learn to tolerate immune-system attacks, adjust to them, and resist them.

However, many types of cancer cells display unusual antigens on their cell membranes that don't belong on that type of cell or that particular tissue. These antigens are specific to a certain type of tumor, so the immune system can recognize cancer cells when that type of tumor is present. One example of such an antigen is glycosphingolipid GD2, which normally only appears in significant amounts on the outer surface membranes of nerve cells, where the blood-brain barrier limits the immune system's ability to attack it. But GD2 is present on the cell surface of several different types of tumors: neuroblastoma, astrocytoma, medulloblastoma, soft-tissue sarcoma, and osteosarcoma. Since the immune system can recognize it in these tumors, GD2 antigen can be used as a tumor-specific target for immunotherapy.

Other tumor cells display cell-surface receptors (a receptor is a specialized protein that recognizes an antigen and binds to it) that are almost always absent on the surface of healthy cells. These receptors activate cellular signals, transmitted by means of a chemical pathway within the cell, that can cause unlimited, uncontrollable growth, division, and multiplication of the cancer cells. A great example is a receptor known as $ErbB_2$, which is produced at high levels on the surface of breast cancer cells. $ErbB_2$ is another example of a target substance for immunotherapy.

There are several types of cancer immunotherapy.

- Monoclonal antibody therapy

- Cancer vaccines (cell-based immunotherapy)

- Immunotherapy using natural products

- Radioimmunotherapy

- Topical immunotherapy

MONOCLONAL ANTIBODY THERAPY

An antibody is a protein produced by white blood cells in response to antigen activity. It binds to the antigen in order to help destroy abnormal cells. Antibodies are an important element in the immune response. They help the immune system recognize foreign antigens and simultaneously stimulate the immune response. A monoclonal antibody is made in a laboratory and is designed to bind to a specific antigen—for example, one of the unusual antigens I described above that are specific to certain tumors. Monoclonal antibody technology thus enables scientists to create antibodies that target individual cancers.

The development of this technology was based on recognition of the importance of antibodies in relation to cancer. The central role played by such antibodies in allergic reactions as hay fever had long been clear, but no one (except for alternative physicians) paid attention to their function in cancer. Once the realization dawned, however, monoclonal antibody technology progressed rapidly, and a number of FDA-approved drugs containing these antibodies came on the market: in 1997, rituximab (Rituxan); in 2004, cetuximab (Erbitux) and bevacizumab (Avastin); and in 2006, panitumumab (Vectibix).

Think about this for a moment: there are plenty of other immuno-stimulating remedies—I listed many of them in Chapter 3—that are not approved by the FDA and never will be. How, then, did the new mono-clonal antibody drugs get approved? It's simple. These are drugs manu-factured by big pharmaceutical companies, which make a huge profit from them. By contrast, natural immune-stimulating remedies bring in only small profits since manufacturing them is cheap—no need to spend millions of dollars creating patented molecules and then putting them through clinical trials. All natural remedies have been used for years, and their success has been demonstrated by successful results with thousands of patients.

So, you might ask, what's wrong with big drug companies making big profits? Nothing at all, especially if their drugs are effective in killing can-cer cells, without major side effects. In fact, though, in addition to being quite costly, these drugs are not that effective. Sometimes they do work, but each drug works for only one, or at most two, types of cancer, and most have considerable side effects.

Table 5.1 introduces you to these monoclonal antibodies.

CANCER VACCINES—CELL-BASED IMMUNOTHERAPY

In my opinion, cancer vaccines are a much more effective treatment for all types of cancer than monoclonal antibody therapy. They have been known and studied for over a century, but their development has been much slower than that of monoclonal antibodies, and most conventional medical experts still consider them an experimental, unproven (or almost unproven) form of immunotherapy. As you will see, the original, very effective cancer vaccine that dates back to the nineteenth century lan-guishes in obscurity, and is actually illegal today in the U.S., while drug companies rush to develop expensive vaccines that may work as well, but not better.

I believe cancer vaccines should be described as cell-based immuno-therapy, since they use immune-system cells, such as cytokines, macro-phages, T cells, or other types of cells that are taken either from the person with cancer or from a donor. These cells are treated in various ways in the lab, then injected back into the patient. Some injected

TABLE 5.1. FDA-APPROVED MONOCLONAL ANTIBODIES

ANTIBODY	BRAND NAME	TARGET ANTIGEN	WHAT IT TREATS
Alemtuzumab	Campath	CD52	Chronic lymphocytic leukemia
Bevacizumab	Avastin	Vascular endothelial growth factor (VEGF)	Breast cancer, colorectal cancer, glioblastoma, kidney cancer, non-small-cell lung cancer
Cetuximab	Erbitux	Epidermal growth factor receptor	Colorectal cancer, head and neck cancer
Denosumab	Xgeva	Rank ligand protein	Cancer spread to bone
Gemtuzumab	Mylotarg	CD33	Acute myelogenous leukemia (used with calicheamicin, an antibiotic)
Ibritumomab tiuxetan	Zevalin	CD20	Non-Hodgkin's lymphoma (used in radioimmunotherapy with the radioactive isotopes yttrium-90 or indium-111)
Ipilimumab	Yervoy	CTLA-4	Melanoma
Ofatumumab	Arzerra	CD20	Chronic lymphocytic leukemia (CLL)
Panitumumab	Vectibix	Epidermal growth factor receptor	Colorectal cancer
Rituximab	Rituxan, Mabthera	CD20	Non-Hodgkin's lymphoma, chronic lymphocytic leukemia (CLL)
Tositumomab	Bexxar	CD20	Non-Hodgkin's lymphoma (used in radioimmunotherapy with the radioactive isotope iodine-131)
Trastuzumab	Herceptin	ErbB2	Breast cancer

immune cells are highly cytotoxic to cancer cells and can destroy them. Other injected cells stimulate the patient's own immune response.

Some vaccines that are referred to as cancer vaccines don't actually target cancer cells. They resemble childhood vaccines for measles, rubella, and other diseases, which are given to prevent disease by using a weakened or killed form of a virus or bacterium to stimulate an immune response specific to that microorganism. An example of such single-purpose vaccines is one used against human papilloma virus (HPV) that helps prevent sexually caused cancers (anal, cervical, vaginal, and vulvar). Another is a hepatitis-B vaccine that may lower the risk of some liver cancers. But these vaccines only target individual microorganisms that can cause cancer or contribute to its development. The goal of true cancer vaccines, on the other hand, is to provide general immunity by stimulating the immune system as a whole to attack cancer that's already present in the body. Real cancer vaccines mean real business: they throw at cancer cells all the immune ammunition that's available. They are a form of active immunotherapy, meaning that they activate the body's immune response to target cancer cells.

Dr. Coley's Discovery

I can't possibly talk about cancer vaccines without mentioning William Coley, M.D., the real pioneer of these vaccines. Coley was a young surgeon at New York Memorial Hospital (now Memorial Sloan-Kettering Cancer Center), who in the early 1890s became dissatisfied with then-existing cancer treatments. After the loss of his very first patient, a seventeen-year-old girl who died two and a half months after he performed surgery on her for bone sarcoma, Coley began a search for a better treatment. He came across the medical record of an immigrant patient with sarcoma of the left cheek. The man had had surgery, but the tumor was so large that the surgeon could not remove all of it. He was also unable to close the huge postoperative wound, and the patient developed a severe wound infection with erysipelas (cellulitis, a skin infection) caused by the bacterium *Streptococcus pyogenes,* which gave him a high fever. To the surprise of his doctors, the man's tumor shrank after each attack of fever, until it was completely gone.

Tracking down this patient, Coley found that he had no signs of cancer and claimed overall excellent health. The only evidence of his former disease was the scar caused by the surgery and infection. The man survived for many decades. His was a typical case of spontaneous tumor regression. Such cases have been known for centuries and are mentioned often in the medical literature. Coley suspected that the patient's infection and fever were both somehow connected to his miraculous recovery.

Deciding to perform a clinical experiment, he infected more than ten cancer patients with live streptococcus erysipelas. Not all of them developed erysipelas, but of those who did, some experienced regression of their tumors. However, two or three others died from the infection, since no antibiotic drugs existed at that time. Coley therefore developed a vaccine made from heat-killed bacteria that would not be strong enough to kill anyone. To make this vaccine he added a second bacterium, *Serratia marcescens,* to the *Streptococcus pyogenes,* in order to produce a synergistic effect. The resulting vaccine became known as Coley's toxins (it has since also been called Coley's vaccine, Coley fluid, and mixed bacterial vaccine). And guess what? Coley's toxins cured many patients—not just those with sarcomas but people with lymphomas, carcinomas, melanomas, and myelomas.

Coley's toxins even helped some patients with terminal cancer. He injected the vaccine directly into the primary tumor site and into metastases, whenever they were accessible. To prevent recurrence, the vaccine was administered several times a week over a minimum of six months. One clear common feature of all successful cases was that the vaccine produced a fever.

Coley's Vaccine and Fever

Coley observed that the most important common denominator of tumor regression was fever. In fact, a retrospective study of patients with inoperable soft-tissue sarcomas who were treated with Coley's vaccine revealed a much better five-year survival rate among those whose fever averaged 38°–40°C (100°–104°F), compared with those whose temperature varied from normal to less than 37°C.

Perhaps Coley's success was less surprising in an age before antibiotic drugs were available to treat infection and fever. Throughout history, physicians had always encouraged development of a fever in order to reinforce the body's immune response to different infections. In fact, the 1927 Nobel Prize in medicine was awarded to Julius Wagner-Jauregg for developing an ingenious method of fever therapy to treat dementia paralytica (neurosyphilis).

Note that fever is a very different animal from hyperthermia. Hyperthermia is a mechanically achieved increase in body temperature that does not produce a systemic immune response, whereas such a response usually does occur in response to a fever triggered by Coley's vaccine. If hyperthermia could cause an immune response, physicians would be using it against all sorts of infections.

Coley's Vaccine and the Immune Connection

With respect to Coley's vaccine's ability to stimulate an immune response, something is known today that Coley did not know—specifically, that introducing his vaccine into the body triggers multiple cytokine cascades. (Cytokines are substances produced by white blood cells that regulate the immune response; they include interleukins, interferons, and tumor-necrosis factor, or TNF. A cascade is a series of chemical reactions.) These cascades in turn set off a multitude of other cascades, as well as a whole range of responses by various cells of the immune system that kill cancer cells. Different cytokines may participate in these cytotoxic cascades.

To give you an idea of how complex these cytokine cascades are, here's a list of the cytokines produced by one of the single-purpose vaccines I referred to above. Bacillus Calmette-Guérin (BCG) contains only one bacterium. In the past it was used worldwide as a vaccine against tuberculosis; now it's used to treat superficial bladder cancer. Unlike Coley's vaccine, BCG is a live vaccine, and it isn't administered to produce a fever. However, the cytokines triggered by these two vaccines are similar.

When BCG is placed directly into a patient's bladder, the following cytokines are detected in the patient's urine: IL-1, IL-2, IL-6, IL-8, IL-10, IL-12, IL-18, interferon-gamma-inducible-protein 10, macrophage colony stimulating factor, and TNF alpha. Don't worry about what the names mean—just note how many cytokines are found after administration of just one bacterium. And Coley's vaccine contains two of them.

What's more, during the entire course of a Coley vaccine treatment, many other cytokines are produced that cause different reactions, ranging from increasing the immune response to decreasing it. And cytokine response is only a tiny part of the entire complex immune connection that results in tumor regression, which involves not just cytokines but monocytes (some of which turn into macrophages that *eat* cancer cells) and dendritic cells, among others. Remember that BCG can only treat bladder cancer, and not even advanced bladder cancer. Successfully attacking advanced invasive cancer requires a powerful response by the entire immune system. That would require a much more potent vaccine, which in the case of BCG can be dangerous, since it's a live vaccine. My conclusion is that in order to create a truly sufficient immune response from a vaccine, it is preferable to use two synergistic killed bacteria. Administering just one won't do the whole job—and cancer needs the whole job and nothing but.

In fact, an analysis of Coley's cases of cancer regression determined that they resulted from a nonspecific immune response. In other words, a successful vaccine against cancer must call up every single one of the immune system's many defensive tactics.

Here is a description of the series of events that results from administration of Coley's vaccine:[2]

- Fever generates inflammatory mediators (the cytokines), which stimulate tissue (inflammation connection).

- Tissue inflammation wakes up resting dendritic cells.

- Dendritic cells activate T cells.

- The fever may also cause physical damage to the cancer cells, which leads them to produce many more antigens. The dendritic cells see these and present them to lymphocytes for execution.

To show you that Coley's vaccine stands up well to scientific investigation, Table 5.2 shows the five-year survival rates of his own treatments. It's based on data collected by Coley's daughter, Helen Coley Nauts, who reviewed her father's charts.

TABLE 5.2. HISTORICAL FIVE-YEAR SURVIVAL RATES AFTER COLEY'S VACCINE		
TYPE OF CANCER	NO. OF PATIENTS	FIVE-YEAR SURVIVAL
Non-Hodgkin's lymphoma	86	42 (49 percent)
Hodgkin's lymphoma	15	19 (67 percent)
Ovarian (nonsurgical—patient did not have surgery)	15	10 (67 percent)
Breast (nonsurgical)	20	13 (65 percent)
Melanoma (nonsurgical)	17	10 (60 percent)
Giant cell sarcoma (nonsurgical)	19	15 (79 percent)

Based on Nauts, H.C., Cancer Research Institute. Monograph #18, 1984.

COLEY'S VACCINE AND THE DANGER MODEL

Coley always insisted that, for optimum effect, his vaccine should be injected every day if the patient could tolerate it, or at least every other day. He observed that discontinuing the vaccine for a few days could lead to regrowth of any residual tumor. Some current research supports the idea that stimulating the immune system not just once or twice, but over a considerable period of time, keeps it in optimal condition to ward off threats.

A 2008 article in *New Scientist* magazine bears the intriguing title "Filthy Healthy: The Cancer Hygiene Hypothesis."[3] *Filth* and *health* don't seem compatible, do they? But as the author, Jessica Marshall, explains, exposure to dirt and the accompanying germs actually seems to help people fight off some types of cancer. Researchers, she says, have been scrambling around the so-called *hygiene hypothesis* for decades, trying to understand why, for example, there is an increased incidence of allergies and asthma in developed countries. The theory is that the absence of various pathogens in our hygienic modern societies means that our immune systems have fewer threats to defend against and therefore get out of whack, resulting in overreactions to stimuli like pollen.

Several studies confirm that exposure to viruses and bacteria does reduce the risk of developing cancer. Ellen Chang of the Northern California Cancer Center in Fremont found that children who attended day-care centers had a reduced risk of developing childhood leukemia and Hodgkin's lymphoma when they became adolescents. Harvey Checkoway of the University of Washington–Seattle examined cancer rates among women who worked at a cotton textile factory in Shanghai and had been exposed to endotoxin (a bacterial toxin found in cotton dust). Workers who were exposed for longer periods and to higher levels of endotoxin had a much lower incidence of many types of cancer—including pancreas, liver, stomach, lung, and breast.

Why get so excited over endotoxin? As Marshall puts it, "The simplest explanation is that exposure to viruses and bacteria—through infections, vaccinations, or proteins such as endotoxin—stimulates the immune system and boosts its anti-cancer activity." That is, keeping the immune system on its toes can not only prevent some cancers but also help get rid of many others once they develop. And this insight goes back to Polly Matzinger and her Danger Model of immunity, which I described in the Prologue.

As noted, the Danger Model proposes that constant stimulation of the immune response by *dangerous elements* (not just viruses and bacteria, but also cancer cells, which play the role of antigens that the immune system attacks) keeps the immune system on constant alert. In effect, the Danger Model confirms the efficacy and the necessity of Coley's vaccine.

In the traditional model of immunity, the immune system discriminates between self and nonself. In the case of cancer, that model says, T and B lymphocytes recognize invasion by cancer cells as a foreign threat and initiate an attack. But cancer cells are like chameleons, disguising themselves in sneaky ways. The immune system becomes unable to see the cancer cell antigens and calls off the attack. It's here that the Danger Model becomes really useful. It suggests that what wakes up the immune system are alarm signals from damaged (cancerous) tissues.

These alarm signals from injured tissues are sent out by cells called antigen-presenting cells (APCs). APCs include macrophages, monocytes, and dendritic cells. Matzinger describes APCs as "sentinels . . . like sleeping sheepdogs" that are awakened by these alarm signals and jump up to protect the flock.[4] APCs then send signals that activate T cells. Usually T cells remain active for only a few days, then die or take a break to rest.

In order to stay active so they can go on the attack when needed, they must receive the signals from APCs. The APCs help the T cells recognize antigens on foreign cells, including cancer cells, by carrying these antigens on their surfaces and presenting them to the T cells.

The Danger Model suggests that effectively killing cancer cells requires repeated stimulation of the immune system (vaccination) with appropriate antigens (danger signals) in order to maintain its awareness that the tumor is a threat. If you only vaccinate once, the immune connection will be broken, the immune response will fade away, the cancer will survive, and the patient will surrender to the disease. Repeated vaccination resends the danger signal, so the immune system stays on constant alert. Matzinger cautions that the immune system must continue to attack until the danger is gone. "If you have a vaccine that makes a tumor get smaller . . . ," she advises, "DON'T STOP! . . . Keep injecting . . . until the last tumor cell is gone."[5] That is why William Coley insisted on daily vaccination until tumor regression was complete. In fact, Polly Matzinger credits her Danger Model concept to Coley.

The current recommendation is to administer Coley's vaccine daily (if possible) for about six months. By that time there should be tumor regression. The sad fact, however, is that Coley's vaccine was effectively banned in this country in 1963, when the FDA assigned it the status of a "new drug." This meant that before it could be used again, it had to go through a long approval process requiring millions of dollars and fifteen to twenty years of clinical trials. At that time there was no one who could take this project on. There is now some hope, however. A small Canadian company, MBVax Bioscience, has developed a version that it calls Coley Fluid. In 2006, the company launched several small limited trials, still ongoing as of this writing. However, its product is available for clinical use only to physicians who practice in countries that allow them to prescribe experimental drugs for use by patients with end-stage disease (the U.S. is one of these countries and allows compassionate use).

Coley's vaccine is available in Mexico, Columbia, the Bahamas, and a few other countries. Many patients go to these countries for their initial treatment with the vaccine. They are then given a supply of vaccine that they self-administer at home. FDA regulations also allow it to be administered by an American physician after the patient has had the initial treatment abroad.

Meanwhile, with Coley's vaccine unavailable, physicians looked for other substances that could stimulate an immune response. One possibility was to administer a single cytokine: TNF, interleukin, or interferon on its own. Unfortunately, it is difficult to reproduce a cytotoxic cascade with single-cytokine therapy because a great many of them are needed to kill cancer.

DENDRITIC CELL VACCINES

Dendritic cells are a type of antigen-presenting cell. Dendritic cell vaccines are made of dendritic cells taken from the blood of a donor, then mixed in the laboratory with tumor cells. The donated dendritic cells can be the patient's own cells (in which case they are known as autologous cells) or from another person (allogeneic cells). The mixed cells are fused into hybrid cells that share the same cell membrane. The result is dendritic cells that have tumor antigens on their surface. These cells are injected into the patient in order to boost the immune system's ability to recognize and destroy the patient's cancer cells.

Most T cells recognize just one specific antigen on the surface of a cell. They attack it by binding to it, then cause it to self-destruct (apoptosis). But, as I've explained, these T cells must be activated before they can destroy cancer cells, and this is the job of the dendritic cells in the vaccine. In effect, the dendritic cell is saying, "Here, I brought you an antigen—finish it off."

Many clinics overseas (in Mexico, the Bahamas, Germany, and elsewhere) prepare their own vaccines and transfuse activated dendritic cells into the bloodstream and tissues of cancer patients. The result is the same cascade of events as in the immune response to Coley's vaccine—showing once again the operation of the Danger Model, as well as the immune connection in action.

Creating Dendritic Cells by Photophoresis

Carole Berger and Richard Edelson at Yale found a way to create dendritic cells overnight. They treated a small amount of a person's blood with a photosensitivity drug and long-wave UV light (UVA). The effect was to convert monocytes (a type of white blood cell) into dendritic cells full of antigens specific to the patient's own tumor.[6] Then they vaccinated the patient with the treated blood. The result was a long-term complete remission of cutaneous T-cell lymphoma in 40 percent of those who were treated.

A few overseas clinics offer this treatment. They have equipment that captures and cultures monocytes into dendritic cells, which are then transfused into the patient's body, enabling the immune system to recognize cancer antigens and activate T lymphocytes to eradicate them—another version of the same mechanism exploited by Coley more than a century ago. Unfortunately, this type of cancer vaccine is only available in Mexico, the Bahamas, and a few other countries.

NOVEL CANCER VACCINES IN THE U.S.

American drug companies are finally catching up with William Coley, and a number of vaccines that stimulate an immune response are either in development or already have FDA approval. At the 2011 meeting of the American Society of Clinical Oncology, several companies reported progress on these so-called novel cancer vaccines—and market researchers are enthusiastically forecasting a huge market for them.

For example, a company called Agenus presented Prophage G-200, which uses heat-shock proteins to send a danger signal to the immune system. In a phase 2 clinical trial, Prophage-G 200 almost doubled the survival time of patients with recurring glioblastoma multiforme. Provenge (sipuleucel-T) is a dendritic cell vaccine that the FDA approved in 2010 for treatment of advanced, hormone-therapy–resistant prostate cancer. In phase 3 trials, Provenge, produced by Dendreon, increased survival by an average of four months, with only mild side effects. However, the three treatments that are needed cost $100,000, leaving many wondering how an already overburdened Medicare system can bear the price.

SEMI-ALLOGENEIC CANCER VACCINES

The cancer vaccines currently available may be exciting, but they also present problems. They don't always stimulate the immune system to mount an effective response, since the T cells don't always recognize the cancer antigens. But new types of dendritic-cell vaccines that are in the works hold some promise. One type is known as semi-allogeneic cancer vaccines.

Semi-allogeneic vaccines avoid the expense and difficulty of creating fully custom-made vaccines by using allogeneic as well as autologous cells to make the hybrid cells, in much the same manner as some dendritic cell vaccines, but by a different technique. In mouse studies, these vaccines protected the treated mice against cancer induced by the researchers, whereas control mice developed tumors. The vaccines induced a high number of cytokines, which means a better immune system response. The vaccines are now in clinical trials. It may be that dendritic cells in semi-allogeneic vaccines may actually be better than fully autologous dendritic cells in inducing anti-tumor effects.

InCVAX—LASER-ASSISTED IMMUNOTHERAPY

INCVAX is a two-step treatment developed by Immunophotonics that makes use of a person's own tumor cells without a complicated lab procedure for preparing them. First, a laser heats the tumor, releasing cancer antigens into the tissue. Then a drug called Protectin is injected around the tumor site. Protectin is made of chitin, which comes from the shells of crustaceans and is said to be nontoxic. It activates APCs and facilitates their interaction with the cancer antigens, which they present to T cells. The result is a systemic immune system response, which according to the company eliminates both the primary tumor and distant metastases in those who respond to the treatment. The treatment takes about an hour, and patients need at most three treatments.

According to their website, the company is preparing an Investigational New Drug (IND) application for FDA approval. However, two studies they conducted abroad showed promising results on patients with breast cancer and melanoma. I am extremely impressed by the concept behind this treatment: it's not painful, it has minimal side effects, and the studies done so far show no evidence of toxicity. Last but not least, it won't be as expensive as any other FDA-approved treatment I've mentioned. So I urge you to be on the alert for news about it.

RADIOIMMUNOTHERAPY

This treatment uses two drugs in the form of conjugated monoclonal antibodies. Conjugating a monoclonal antibody means joining it to another substance, in this case a radioactive particle. The monoclonal antibody acts as the carrier that takes the radioactive particle to the target antigen, where the radioactivity can destroy it. Most of the research on radioimmunotherapy is limited to lymphoma, since that form of cancer is highly radiosensitive. This treatment is used when a patient's cancer has not responded to standard treatment.

- Ibritumomab tiuxetan links a monoclonal antibody to yttrium-90 or indium-111. It's used to treat B cell non-Hodgkin's lymphoma.

- Tositumomab links a different monoclonal antibody to iodine-131. This drug is used mainly in those with relapsed follicular lymphoma.

I have not used radioimmunotherapy in my own practice. I think it's a great idea that represents an integration of radiation and immunotherapy. But much work remains to be done to improve and widen the horizons of this treatment, especially to discover whether it can be used for other types of cancers.

TOPICAL IMMUNOTHERAPY

Topical refers to a particular surface area, in this case the skin. Topical immunotherapy is used mainly by dermatologists to treat benign and malignant skin tumors. It involves an immune-enhancement cream (Imiquimod) that stimulates production of interferon, which causes the patient's own T cells to destroy warts, basal cell carcinoma, squamous cell carcinoma, cutaneous T-cell lymphoma, and superficial spreading melanoma. Topical immunotherapy has only a few applications, but it's quite useful for those.

NATURAL-PRODUCT IMMUNOTHERAPY

In Chapter 3 I've already described quite a few natural products that stimulate an immune response—such as vitamin C, Zadaxin, and

Iscador—and in Chapter 8 you'll read about more of them, including Avemar, Poly-MVA, and the entire family of mushrooms containing beta-glucan. Natural-product immunotherapy has a huge place in this book, since it's the driving force behind the entire complex program of integrative cancer therapy.

Natural-product immunotherapy can be used as a treatment on its own or, preferably, in conjunction with conventional and other alternative treatments as a player in the entire integrative/alternative orchestra. By now you probably can tell me why it's preferable to use so many therapies: because to treat cancer successfully, it is important to address all the cancer connections.

FINAL THOUGHTS

Seeing the conventional oncology establishment participating in a paradigm shift toward cancer immunotherapy makes me extremely happy and excited. It's about time this happened. Cancer is a vicious animal that must be dealt with accordingly, not only by killing it with outside forces (the conventional trio) but also by enlisting the most mysterious, powerful system inside the body where this animal resides: the immune system.

Of course, cutting out a tumor or zapping it with radiation is a much simpler method for treating cancer. But you never know when residual cancer cells remain lurking within the body, more than happy to multiply and spread, given that the immune system is not on high alert so there's no surveillance from within. That's why the immune therapies are irreplaceable—especially the cancer vaccines.

If the late Dr. Coley could return and observe the state of cancer treatment today, I think he'd be both thrilled and sad. He'd be delighted to learn that oncologists and oncology researchers have at last accepted his concept of cancer vaccination. And I'm sure he wouldn't care whether conventional or alternative practitioners were using his vaccine concept, as long as they helped their patients. Coley would be quite proud and pleased to find that Polly Matzinger's Danger Model of immunity had partly solved the puzzle of why his vaccine worked, and that most of the mechanisms underlying its success were uncovered with the discovery of cytokines and their cascades, especially type-1 interferon in 1957 and

TNF-alpha in 1968. He'd also be happy to learn that many other types of cancer vaccines have been developed and that their use has become increasingly popular. And he'd rejoice to learn that MBVax Bioscience was conducting clinical trials in order once again to prove the efficacy of Coley's vaccine.

But Coley would certainly be sad to find that his vaccine was still banned by the FDA and that his fever concept had never achieved the status it deserves as a great immune booster. He would be distressed to realize that even though almost half a century has passed since the discovery of interferon, cancer vaccines have not advanced as far as they could have if they had received proper attention, so that his own vaccine, developed in the 1890s, remains unsurpassed for treating cancer.

I take comfort in the fact that Coley's legacy is still very much alive, and I'm sure that cancer vaccines—and Coley's vaccine in particular—will have a long and fruitful life in the future.

CHAPTER 6

─ ─ ─ ─ ─

Oxidative Therapies—
Oxygen in Action

INITIAL THOUGHTS

Whenever I begin writing a new chapter, I think: What's special about this topic? Naturally, I asked myself this question as I began writing about oxygen.

Oxidative therapies (the correct scientific name; many people call them oxygen therapies, as I will here) are indeed special. I cherish these treatments; they're quite dear to my heart. In fact, in 2003 I published a book titled *Oxygen to the Rescue,* which described how integrative physicians use oxygen therapies to heal a wide range of diseases and conditions. Cancer played a relatively small role in that book, so this one fills in the blanks and explains how these therapies help heal cancer.

Oxygen comprises 21 percent of the air we breathe. It's abundant and cheap, and years of clinical experience plus many research studies have demonstrated that it's a safe, effective therapeutic agent. So you might imagine that using it to treat a whole range of chronic degenerative diseases, including cancer, would be considered quite logical and reasonable. After all, Dr. Otto Warburg, who discovered that cancer cells metabolize sugar instead of oxygen (*see* Prologue), said, "The prime cause of cancer is the replacement of normal oxygen respiration of body cells by an anaerobic [lacking in oxygen] cell respiration." So anything that gets more oxygen into those cells should be good, right? Unfortunately, as you will see, logic and reason do not rule the conventional attitude toward oxygen therapies.

BASICS OF OXYGEN THERAPIES

Oxygen therapies (also known as bioxidative therapies) are a crucial component of an integrative cancer treatment program. To explain what these therapies are and how they work, I must first define a few terms.

- *Oxidation* is a chemical reaction in which an atom or molecule loses electrons—that is, they are transferred to another atom or molecule. Oxidation occurs when oxygen combines with another substance, changing the nature of both. It's the most important process that results from breathing because it enables the body to function properly. But, as discussed in the Prologue, it can also be a destructive process when free radicals steal electrons from stable molecules, causing cell damage.

- *Reduction* is a chemical reaction in which an atom gains electrons from another atom. Oxidation and reduction together are essential for maintaining the body's chemical balance.

- *Oxygenation* is the process of increasing the amount of oxygen in blood or tissues.

Oxygen therapies are essentially methods for oxygenating the body. It is important to get oxygen into tissues because it promotes the body's healing capacity and can also kill various microbes, as well as, in some cases, cancer cells. These therapies play an absolutely invaluable supporting role in cancer treatment, for they can stop cancer's growth. I consider them an essential component of an integrative anti-cancer program.

Oxygenating the body is a simple enough concept. But critics of these very valuable therapies oppose them on the ground that they produce large numbers of free radicals that will cause cell damage and mutations. Here I must apologize, but this makes me laugh. Aren't free radicals said to be part of what makes chemo and radiation so effective? And don't conventional oncologists warn against taking antioxidants lest they diminish the beneficial effects of these same free radicals? So how do free radicals suddenly become dangerous when they result from oxygen therapies?

In fact, oxygen therapies *don't* produce large amounts of free radicals. They produce some, but not enough to cause damage. And in any case, integrative physicians don't use oxygen therapies because they create free radicals. They use these therapies because oxygen devastates cancer cells. The sections below explain the benefits of what I like to call the Fantastic Four: Hydrogen peroxide therapy, ozone therapy, ultraviolet irradiation of blood (UVIB), and hyperbaric oxygen therapy (HBOT)

FANTASTIC #1—HYDROGEN PEROXIDE THERAPY

Most people know hydrogen peroxide as a colorless liquid that they buy in the drugstore and keep in the medicine cabinet to use as a disinfectant or antiseptic, as a mouthwash, or for bleaching hair. But hydrogen peroxide is much more than this. Charles Farr, M.D., Ph.D., a brilliant researcher, spent many years conducting clinical work with hydrogen peroxide, which led to his nomination in 1993 for the Nobel Prize in Medicine. It's due to Dr. Farr that hydrogen peroxide is available as a treatment, and I am immensely proud that I received my own basic knowledge of hydrogen peroxide use from him personally.

Once you know the actual physiological effects hydrogen peroxide has on the body, you'll understand its value for undoing many of the evils caused by cancer. Because it's administered by intravenous infusion, hydrogen peroxide gets into the circulatory system right away. Let's follow what happens to hydrogen peroxide once it enters the body.

The hydrogen peroxide molecule consists of two hydrogen atoms and two oxygen atoms. When it hits the blood, it splits into a water molecule (two hydrogen atoms plus one oxygen atom) and an oxygen molecule that consists of a single oxygen atom, called singlet oxygen. The standard and most stable form of oxygen is a molecule consisting of two oxygen atoms (O_2), whereas singlet oxygen is a powerful oxidizing agent and is mainly responsible for hydrogen peroxide's multiple therapeutic properties. Chemically the hydrogen peroxide–blood reaction looks like this:

$$H_2O_2 \longrightarrow H_2O + O$$

When hydrogen peroxide gets into the bloodstream, it is greeted by two enzymes: catalase and cytochrome C. As explained in Chapter 3, the function of catalase is to convert hydrogen peroxide into water and singlet oxygen. Catalase goes to work immediately, but it doesn't convert all the hydrogen peroxide that's present. It leaves part of that hydrogen peroxide for cytochrome C, which binds with it to form a complex. After this complex has been circulating in the blood for about forty minutes, cytochrome C acts like catalase and splits the hydrogen peroxide into water and singlet oxygen. During this forty minutes, the circulating blood delivers the hydrogen peroxide/cytochrome cancer complex to every cell in the body. Not a single cell is missed. So when cytochrome C does split the hydrogen peroxide, oxygen is released inside every cell, oxygenating every tissue in the body.

THE GOOD DEEDS OF SINGLET OXYGEN

If singlet oxygen is the powerful weapon hidden inside hydrogen peroxide, what does it do once it's inside the cells? For normal cells, it brings health by increasing their ability to heal any damage. But for cancerous cells, the story is totally different.

- Cancer cells cannot stand oxygen, singlet oxygen included. The same is true of viruses, bacteria, and fungi, those friends and accomplices of cancer that so frequently infect people with cancer. Singlet oxygen kills these accomplices by oxidizing them. It also decreases the cancer cells' aggressiveness.

- Singlet oxygen also oxidizes toxins and biological waste products (the normal outputs of such various body functions as metabolism), transforming them into inert substances. This action enables the kidneys and liver to detoxify the body and eliminate waste products much more easily.

- Singlet oxygen increases metabolism in the mitochondria in every healthy cell, which also helps the body detoxify.

- Singlet oxygen boosts the immune system: first, by stimulating production of T-helper cells, and second, by encouraging the activity of interferon-gamma, a type of cytokine with immune-stimulating activity (immune connection).

- Singlet oxygen decreases the inflammation that is so often present during the development of cancer (inflammation connection).

- Singlet oxygen mimics the actions of insulin. Chapter 4 discusses what insulin means for cancer cells—it means problems.

- Because singlet oxygen dissolves cholesterol, it can be used to treat atherosclerosis (hardening of the arteries, which involves cholesterol buildup), and also to correct MID (MID connection). Decreased blood cholesterol levels lead to decreased cholesterol in T lymphocytes. Cholesterol in T lymphocytes affects them like cataracts: it impairs their ability to see cancer cell antigens. Removing the cholesterol improves their vision. The result is better immune function.

Thus, simple-seeming singlet oxygen turns out to be the secret ingredient of hydrogen peroxide therapy. It addresses five cancer connections—the oxygen connection, the sugar connection, the immune connection, the MID connection, and the inflammatory connection.

MORE ON HYDROGEN PEROXIDE AND CANCER

Were you aware that large sea creatures (dolphins, whales, sharks) never get cancer? They all swim in seawater, which is full of hydrogen peroxide. The same benefit is available to humans. In 1858, a young girl saw a vision of the Virgin Mary in a grotto in the village of Lourdes, in southwest France. Pilgrims have traveled there ever since to drink and bathe in the water that flows from a spring in the sanctuary, which is said to have healing powers. Miraculous cures have been reported. But in my opinion it's not the miraculous power of the Virgin that's behind the healing properties of the water. That water is loaded with hydrogen peroxide, which can enter the body through the skin.

And you don't have to go to Lourdes to bathe in hydrogen-peroxide-enriched water. Just fill your bathtub with water and pour in a pint of food-grade (35 percent) hydrogen peroxide. Many people with arthritis swear by these baths, because they reduce inflammation. Cancer patients can enjoy them during radiation therapy and chemo. They'll certainly appreciate how they feel energized and less toxic afterward.

As a cancer therapy, hydrogen peroxide is usually administered intravenously, in a solution of 250cc of normal saline or sterile water to 3cc of pharmaceutical grade (3 percent) hydrogen peroxide. This treatment takes forty-five minutes. Alternatively, the physician may use 5cc of 3 percent hydrogen peroxide in 500cc of normal saline or sterile water, administered over one and a half hours. Patients usually tolerate hydrogen peroxide treatment very well. I see them leave the office energetic and happy, since they feel so much better afterward.

How safe is the therapy? Since the 1980s, over 7,700 articles related to hydrogen peroxide have been published in conventional medical journals. These reports indicate that hydrogen peroxide has very few side effects. Occasionally someone may experience vein irritation and (rarely) vein sclerosis (hardening) in reaction to the IV infusion.

I don't advocate hydrogen peroxide therapy as a cancer treatment on its own. But every single one of my cancer patients gets hydrogen peroxide IV treatments as part of my whole program, which also includes vitamin C/K infusions, IPT treatments, various other treatments described in Chapter 3, and of course the other members of the Fantastic Four.

Given how cheap hydrogen peroxide is, why is it practically invisible as a treatment? You probably already know the answer—it can't be patented, which means there are no big profits to be made from it, which means the pharmaceutical industry has no interest in funding research on it. I rest my case.

FANTASTIC #2—
OZONE THERAPY, AN OXIDIZING WEAPON

For years, the medical establishment has unjustly beat up on ozone therapy and made it the subject of heated controversy. Ozone was said to be toxic to the human body, and using it, even researching it, was prohibited. It was such a taboo that instead of saying the word *ozone* out loud, people whispered it. As a consequence, ozone's therapeutic value was never explored scientifically. Yet I've never heard a satisfactory, logical, scientific explanation of why ozone was made a second-class citizen. And if you look at the history of its discovery and medicinal use, you can't deny its tremendous health benefits.

Ozone was discovered by the chemist Christian Friedrich Schönbein in 1840 and first used in 1856 to disinfect operating rooms and sterilize surgical instruments. By the end of the nineteenth century, ozone was used widely in Europe to disinfect drinking water. In 1885, the Florida Medical Association published a description of the therapeutic use of ozone by Charles J. Kenworthy, M.D., of Jacksonville. In 1892, the British medical journal *The Lancet* reported the use of ozone therapy to treat tuberculosis. In 1916, an article by a military surgeon in the same journal reported the successful use of ozone to treat twenty-one cases of war wounds. But after that, there was little research on ozone until 2000, when a group of researchers affiliated with the Scripps Research Institute came up with evidence disputing the main accusation against ozone.[1]

Ozone therapy involves drawing blood from a vein, infusing ozone into it, then returning it to the body, a process known as *autohemotherapy*. For years, this procedure was said to be dangerous, on the ground that infusing ozone into human blood produced free radicals that would oxidize (that is, damage) blood cells and other tissues. The Scripps researchers investigated whether ozone damaged the enzymes in red blood cells, and concluded that those cells were unaffected by ozone. They encouraged clinical trials on the use of ozone autohemotherapy. No such studies were done in the U.S., but research conducted in Canada, Israel, Italy, Japan, and Poland subsequently confirmed that ozone therapy is nontoxic and has no significant side effects.[2]

WHAT OZONE DOES

Basically, ozone therapy is a way to get a great deal of oxygen into the body quickly. Ozone is a colorless gas that surrounds the planet, protecting all living things from the damaging effects of the sun's ultraviolet rays. It's a relatively unstable molecule consisting of three oxygen atoms (chemical symbol O_3). Like hydrogen peroxide, ozone is an oxidizer. But its instability, which is the basis of most of the attacks on it, actually underlies its healing power. Only a minute or two after they're administered, some of the ozone molecules interact with each other to produce stable O_2 molecules. Two molecules of ozone create three molecules of oxygen, as follows:

$$O_3 + O_3 \longrightarrow 3\,O_2$$

This process, in which oxidation and reduction happen simultaneously, is known as dismutation. Because ozone dismutates at a rate of 50 percent every thirty to forty-five minutes, it must be used quickly.

The rest of the ozone that's administered produces hydrogen peroxide, which immediately interacts with amino acids and lipids that are present, forming substances called *ozonides*. The highly reactive ozonide molecules are mainly responsible for the numerous healing effects of ozone therapy.

- Ozonides increase oxygen utilization.

- Ozonides boost the function of the mitochondria, increasing production of ATP and acetyl coenzyme A (acetyl-CoA, a molecule important in oxidation) by about 40 percent, which means you have much more energy. Plus, you want your mitochondria to work optimally, since low-performing mitochondria play a major role in the development of chronic degenerative diseases, including cancer.

- Ozonides increase the ability of antioxidants to neutralize free radicals, protecting against the excessive free-radical formation caused by chemo and radiation.

- Ozonides accelerate glycolysis (the breakdown of sugars). When glycolysis is rapid, glucose is used up quickly. Cancer cells lose their food, and healthy cells burn more oxygen, instead of sugar. They thus increase the release of O_2 from hemoglobin into the tissues, and then into the cancer.

- Ozonides strengthen immune defenses in two ways. They increase production of white blood cells, thereby multiplying the immune system's army of protective cells. Ozonides also stimulate phagocytosis (engulfing of foreign invaders by macrophages).

- Just like Coley's vaccine (see Chapter 5), ozonides support production of the whole range of cytokines (IL-1, IL-2, IL-6, IL-8, IL-10, interferon gamma and beta, GM-CSF [granulocyte-macrophage colony-stimulating factor], TNF-alpha, and TNF beta).

- Ozonides stimulate the function of the reticuloendothelial system (RES), a group of phagocytotic cells that create red and white blood cells and remove harmful materials such as microorganisms and tumor cells from the blood.

• Ozonides have a powerful ability to kill bacteria, viruses, and fungi.

• Ozonides assist the body's anti-inflammatory response by calming inflammatory cytokines.

What an incredibly impressive list, underlining the tremendous healing powers of ozone therapy. What's more, many ozonides last days or even weeks, so their therapeutic effects continue well past the therapy session. And the scope of ozone's healing power is broad, ranging from infectious diseases to circulatory problems, arthritic conditions, and immune disorders. It's truly an anti-aging boon.

OZONE IN CANCER TREATMENT

In cancer specifically, ozone works in several ways.

Ozone Inhibits Cancer-Cell Growth

A number of researchers report that cancer cells cannot handle the number of free radicals produced by ozone, whereas normal cells welcome the extra oxygen. An important lab study published in the journal *Science* in 1980 found that ozone inhibited the growth of cancer cells yet had no dangerous effects on healthy cells.

No clinical studies of ozone as a cancer treatment have been done in the U.S., but in 2004 a group of Spanish researchers reported the results of human trials of ozone therapy. Nineteen patients with incurable head and neck cancer received radiation therapy in conjunction with either tegafur (a chemo drug) or ozone therapy. Those who received ozone were older and had larger, more advanced tumors, but this group survived slightly longer than the group that got chemo. "Ozone therapy can produce an improvement in blood flow and oxygenation in some tissues," the authors concluded.[3] This result ought to encourage many more clinical trials worldwide; but sadly, I haven't noticed any.

It Relieves the Side Effects of Chemo and Radiation

Ozone relieves many of the debilitating problems caused by conventional chemo and radiation. The same Spanish group mentioned above reported healing bladder inflammation caused by radiation (which results in blood in the urine) by inserting distilled water infused with ozone into the bladder.[4] Three Cuban studies on rats reported that ozone therapy helped ward off the adverse effects of the chemo drug cisplatin, which can cause acute kidney damage. Russian researchers came up with similar results with human subjects. They divided fifty-two women with breast cancer into two groups. The thirty-two women in the first group were treated with chemotherapy combined with ozone therapy. The twenty women in the second group received chemo only. The investigators concluded that ozone therapy diminished the chemo drug's effect of suppressing healthy cell growth, improved the patients' quality of life and immune status, and significantly boosted their antioxidant defenses.[5]

It Increases the Effectiveness of Chemo and Radiation

Ozone therapy makes the conventional duo more effective by adding additional oxidative stress. It also decreases cancer cells' resistance to chemo—making it extremely useful as an auxiliary therapy for IPT.

It Kills Cancer Cells

Ozone kills cancer cells on direct contact and successfully treats anal cancers when it is insufflated into the rectum (*see* "How Ozone Is Administered" below).

Ozone and the Cancer Connection

Looking at the many effects of ozonides listed above, it should be pretty clear how ozone addresses these cancer connections: oxygen, immune system, sugar, and inflammation. So you can see why ozone therapy is a vital component of integrative cancer treatment.

How Ozone Is Administered

Ozone can be administered in a variety of ways.

- *Major autohemotherapy transfusions.* This is the most commonly used procedure. 100–250 ml of blood is drawn from a vein, exactly as is done for a blood donation. The blood is then infused with a combination of ozone and oxygen and retransfused into the patient from the IV bag. The procedure takes thirty to forty-five minutes.

- *Minor autohemotherapy transfusion.* In this procedure, only 10 ml of blood is drawn, then treated with the ozone/oxygen mix, and injected into the patient's buttock.

- *Rectal insufflation.* An oxygen/ozone gas mixture is administered through a rectal probe, as in an enema.

- *Bladder insufflation.* An ozone/oxygen solution is inserted into the urinary bladder through a catheter.

- *Ozone sauna.* The patient sits in a steam room, and the ozone/oxygen combination is pumped in along with the steam. Note: breathing in *clean* ozone in unpolluted air is not harmful.

- *Ozonated oil.* The ozone/oxygen combination is infused into olive oil and applied to the skin as a salve to treat skin conditions, such as fungus, that cancer patients are prone to developing. Occasionally, this mixture is also used to treat skin cancer.

- *Ozone plus ultraviolet.* A recently developed method combines ozone with ultraviolet radiation of blood (UVIB). This brilliant idea is discussed in the next section.

RESPONSE TO CRITICS OF OZONE THERAPY

I want to answer conventional medicine's two charges against ozone—that it is a foreign substance, toxic to the body, and that it creates damaging free radicals.

First, ozone is actually produced by the human body. Studies by Scripps Institute researchers have suggested that ozone is naturally produced by human neutrophils (a type of white blood cell). These researchers also discovered that ozone can also be produced in atherosclerotic arteries in response to inflammation. The fact that the human body itself generates ozone indicates that ozone is not foreign to the body, and not toxic.

Second, ozone itself does not produce free radicals. When the pH of its surroundings is lower than 8—that is, acidic—the ozone molecule has a charge that attracts unpaired electrons. By attracting these electrons, the ozone molecules actually eliminate free radicals in the blood and tissues. And let me reassure you that a pH *greater* than 8 has never been found in the human body. In other words, there's nothing to worry about. It's true that the oxygen in the mixture does produce some free radicals, but not very many—and no more than the ozone is able to get rid of.

FANTASTIC #3—THE REMARKABLE TALE OF UVIB

Ultraviolet irradiation of blood (UVIB) sounds like a treatment Dr. McCoy might use in *Star Trek,* but far from being futuristic, it dates back over a century. First discovered by Johann Wilhelm Ritter in 1801, ultraviolet (UV) light was initially investigated in terms of how sunlight affected health. In 1903, Niels Ryberg Finsen received the Nobel Prize in Physiology or Medicine for his use of UV light to treat 300 patients suffering from lupus vulgaris. His work was based on the previous discovery that sunlight could kill bacteria. And in fact, UV light has long been used as a disinfectant.

The first to use UVIB was Kurt Naswitis, who in 1922 directly irradiated blood with UV light through a shunt (small tube). In 1928, Emmet Knott irradiated the blood of a woman with a post-abortion bloodstream infection, saving her life. He later received patents for a UVIB apparatus he invented. Other physicians began to experiment with UVIB and found that it was a remarkable vehicle to cure infection. But then UVIB was abandoned in the wave of enthusiasm over the introduction of antibiotics in the 1950s. What a shame.

It was during the 1970s in Russia—during the same period I was a medical student—that UVIB treatments began to be explored again. In those same years, Richard L. Edelson at Yale University developed a new form of blood irradiation that he named photopheresis. Edelson used it to achieve better results from chemotherapy. Despite the prohibitive cost (about $2,000 per treatment), he treated about 900 patients a year. In 1992, Dr. William Campbell Douglass published his book *Into the Light*, which described all the wonders of hydrogen peroxide and UVIB and was responsible for increasing awareness of UVIB's multiple healing properties.

UVIB was used to treat cancer as early as the 1960s, when Dr. Robert C. Olney, a pioneer of this therapy, reported successfully treating cases of malignant melanoma, metastatic colon cancer, thyroid cancer, and uterine cancer with UVIB. William Campbell Douglas reported successful treatment of metastatic breast and stomach cancers that had spread to the bones and brain. He concluded that UVIB extended the patient's life and significantly improved its quality.

How UVIB Works

UVIB is used mainly as an adjuvant therapy. The treatment is simple. A small amount of blood is drawn from a vein and passed through a machine that exposes it to UV light. UVIB's healing effects all arise from UV light's incredible ability to increase the blood level of oxygen. Although no one really knows exactly *how* this happens, they do know it happens because it increases the amount of oxygen that the hemoglobin contains.

- Increased blood oxygen helps eradicate multiple pathogens. And when oxygen enters the cancer cells, it suffocates them. It may not kill them completely, but it certainly brings them close to death.

- UVIB also attacks microbes directly by triggering chemical reactions that make microbial cell membranes more permeable, thus marking them for death by the cytotoxic T cells. In fact, bacteria, viruses, and most other antibiotic-resistant microorganisms succumb to UVIB treatment.

- Increasing blood oxygen stimulates the cytokine cascade. Therefore, UVIB treatment also has immune and anti-inflammatory effects.

UVIB and the Cancer Connections

- *Oxygen connection.* UVIB increases the concentration of oxygen in the blood.

- *Immune connection.* UVIB increases production of all the foot soldiers of the immune army.

- *Inflammation connection.* UVIB's anti-inflammatory power treats arthritis, bursitis, iritis, pancreatitis, and other inflammatory processes. UVIB also stimulates production of, and activates, corticosteroids and other anti-inflammatory hormones.

Bad News, Good News, and Better News

The bad news is that, because there are as yet only a few sketchy scientific reports of UVIB's anti-cancer properties, it is still considered experimental as a treatment for cancer. But the good news is that anti-cancer use of UVIB is gaining momentum.

Even better news is on the horizon—a new, simple method that combines ozone and UVIB. The person's blood is collected from a vein and an ozone/oxygen mixture is added to it. This ozonated blood is put in the IV bag with normal saline solution and drips back into the vein, passing through a small device that irradiates it with UV—rather like buy one, get another free. Indeed, you get two excellent treatments at once, making this technique doubly effective.

When I first heard about this technique, I said to myself, "As always, any great discovery is essentially a simple one." What a terrific addition to the family of the Fantastic Four. I call it the *Fantastic 4 1/2.*

My own conclusion is also simple: integrative cancer specialists should use UVIB to treat all cancer patients. Conventional oncologists should use it too, although that will take longer to happen. But in over fifty years of research with humans, physicians worldwide have conducted over 300,000 clinical tests affirming the validity of this remarkable therapy, and not a single person was lost. There were no toxic effects, no side effects. Draw your own conclusions.

FANTASTIC #4—HYPERBARIC OXYGEN THERAPY

You have probably heard many stories of potential victims of drowning or carbon monoxide poisoning saved with hyperbaric oxygen therapy (HBOT)—a treatment in which pure oxygen under pressure (pressurized

O_2) is administered inside a special chamber. The history of HBOT goes back at least to the seventeenth century, when a British physician named Henshaw built a special chamber called a domicilium that he pressurized using a bellows. He believed that this treatment could improve digestion and respiration.

HBOT was developed for commercial use in 1935. Best known for its usefulness in treating divers who get decompression illness (the bends), it's also widely used in mainstream medicine to treat carbon monoxide poisoning, poorly healed wounds, and other conditions. Alternative physicians find it beneficial in cases of arthritis, cancer, cerebral palsy, HIV, Lyme disease, multiple sclerosis, optic neuritis, and strokes.

A hyperbaric chamber is either a long cylinder with a transparent top that one person lies down in or a room that accommodates a number of people who breathe in pressurized oxygen through a mask or hood. An HBOT treatment lasts an hour and a half to two hours, with the patient breathing pure oxygen that is pressurized to between 1.5 and 2.5 ATA (ATA is a diving measure of pressure at a specific depth of water; 1 ATA equals atmospheric pressure and 2 ATA equals pressure at thirty-three feet down).

As might be expected, using HBOT as a cancer therapy didn't happen without controversy. Many chemo drugs act by cutting the oxygen supply to the tumor, and HBOT was accused of promoting the proliferation and spread of cancer because it improves nourishment of tumors by promoting angiogenesis (new blood-vessel formation). However, numerous published reports since 1967 suggest that is not the case, since they found no cancer-promoting effects of HBOT. Mice implanted with S-180 sarcoma lived longer, with less tumor growth, when treated with HBOT. And one group of researchers who treated humans with HBOT reported a significant *decrease* in metastases. In that study, HBOT improved disease-free survival for 104 patients with head and neck cancer.[6] In a controlled trial in which 1,500 people with different types of cancers (bladder, bronchus, cervical, head and neck) received HBOT treatments, there was no increase in metastases. Overall, nineteen randomized, controlled trials involving a total of 2,286 patients concluded that HBOT actually reduced mortality from head and neck cancer.

As I've explained, the notion that starving tumors of oxygen promotes tumor growth may not be correct. There is some research indicating that chemo drugs inhibit cancer growth initially, but then promote more invasive cancer growth, sometimes with increased metastasis. That is, the tumor responds to starvation induced by the drugs by becoming more aggressive.[7] This is another reason for the emerging idea that preventing angiogenesis may not be the best treatment. In fact, the blood vessels created by angiogenesis will deliver oxygen to the cancer cells—and you know now what oxygen means for a cancer cell.

"The crucial role that oxygen plays in killing tumors has been underappreciated," noted Bruce Fenton, associate professor of radiation oncology at the Wilmot Cancer Center. He suggested that without oxygen the effects of radiation and chemo may fall short, since cancer cells can often repair themselves. And cancer cells containing oxygen are about two to three times more susceptible to radiation than cells without proper oxygenation.

Paul Okunieff, M.D., head of Radiation Oncology at the Wilmot Cancer Center, University of Rochester, summed up the pro-angiogenesis position: "The tumor is meaner if it's hypoxic [oxygen-starved]. Oxygen is by far the most powerful molecule for making cells vulnerable to radiation. Tumor cells that survive hypoxic conditions are often the cells that are most aggressive, most hardy, and most likely to go out and start new cancer colonies." He added that these cells are also prone to undergo mutations that make them likely to spread.[8] I tend to agree that angiogenesis may be of benefit by bringing oxygen to cancer cells. But that won't be known for sure until more research is done.

HBOT and the Cancer Connections

- *Oxygen connection.* Breathing in 100 percent oxygen under pressure allows extra oxygen to enter the bloodstream and be delivered to every cell in the body. HBOT increases the blood's ability to transport oxygen, and this extra oxygen creates mayhem in the cancer tumor and its cells. The extra oxygen also aids healing of tissues damaged by cancer or radiation.

- *Immune connection.* HBOT augments the immune system's ability to fight the cancer itself and the infections that often accompany it.

- *Inflammation connection.* HBOT helps reduce any inflammatory processes caused either by cancer itself or by radiation therapy.

MIXING AND MATCHING THE FANTASTIC FOUR

Should cancer patients use all four oxygen therapies? My answer is a qualified yes.

Hydrogen peroxide and ozone therapy are *not* substitutes for each other and should be alternated. Ozone therapy is more potent, and usually involves no more than ten treatments two to three times a year. Hydrogen peroxide, on the other hand, can be given two or three times a week for an unlimited period. It's also less expensive than ozone.

Now that the ozone/UVIB treatment combo is available, I suggest that, instead of getting these therapies separately, you use the combined treatment, and alternate it with hydrogen peroxide therapy.

HBOT treatments are surprisingly inexpensive in an office setting, but since the chambers are very costly to buy and maintain, few doctors have them. If you can find a doctor who offers HBOT, you should definitely have this treatment. But if HBOT isn't available, hydrogen peroxide and the ozone/UVIB combo are the way to go.

FINAL THOUGHTS

Only in the environmentally pristine garden of Eden would humans breathe perfectly clean air, full of the optimal amount of oxygen for our bodies. Believe me, the word *cancer* would not exist there. But living here in an industrialized, polluted world where the air never contains sufficient oxygen, people are getting sick, especially with cancer. Faced with this situation, the clever human mind found a variety of ways to deliver extra amounts of this much-needed element to the deprived human body. Thus did the Fantastic Four appear in the world of oncology.

As I've noted, few clinical studies of these wonderful therapies exist, purely because they aren't patentable, and therefore not profitable. Which leads me to ask the pharmaceutical and medical industries: How much is human life worth to you?

Putting my feelings aside, though, I must remind you that there is no scientific evidence showing that oxygen therapy actually kills cancer, except in a few cases, such as the application of ozone directly to anal cancer tumors. Nevertheless, the Fantastic Four are an essential part of integrative anti-cancer treatment. Let me summarize.

- Oxygen therapies make chemotherapy more successful by increasing the sensitivity of cancer cells to chemo drugs. They also help fend off many of chemo's side effects.

- Oxygen therapies improve the efficacy of radiation therapy and help restore the functioning of healthy tissues damaged by radiation.

- Oxygen therapies make IPT much more effective. I firmly believe that they should always be used in conjunction with IPT.

- Finally, these therapies make other alternative treatments (cancer vaccines, vitamin C infusions, and all the other treatments described in Chapter 3) more effective.

That's why I say flatly that every person with cancer who is treated by an integrative physician should have every one of these treatments.

CHAPTER 7

— — — — —

Off-Label Use of Drugs

INITIAL THOUGHTS

Reading the title of this chapter, you may wonder: Why is this alternative physician suddenly talking about drugs? You'd be even more puzzled if you knew that conventional physicians in mainstream oncology departments *don't* talk about the drug treatments this chapter will describe. On the surface, this may make little sense. But a deeper look presents quite a different picture.

The key is in the phrase *off-label use,* which means using these drugs for a purpose other than the one they were originally developed for or (most important) were approved for by the FDA. Off-label use has several serious implications.

- First, the drugs I'll be describing here can't be marketed for their off-label use by their manufacturers.

- Second, off-label use gives insurance carriers a great excuse not to pay claims for prescriptions of these drugs.

- Last but not least, if off-label use results in any known side effects, watch out: the prescribing physician is legally responsible for deviating from *standards of care.* And who wants that headache? Certainly not conventional oncologists.

All this is true even though a great deal of scientific evidence indicates that off-label use of drugs offers tremendous benefits for cancer treatment. So what about patients whose pain can be alleviated by such use?

Who's thinking about them? You can guess: integrative alternative physicians are. What's more, they're doing so without any financial rewards, since they charge patients exactly the same whether drugs are prescribed for the approved use or the off-label use. The fact is, they'll prescribe anything—and I mean anything—that works . . . and only if it works. And that's my own formula for cancer treatment.

You may ask yourself why the pharmaceutical companies aren't promoting off-label use of their drugs? So doing would broaden the applications of their drugs, and they could sell more. However, it would require launching expensive new research for each off-label use—and if the patent on the drug has expired, other companies could sell the drug too. This situation leaves integrative physicians with plenty of enthusiasm, but no support from the medical community or the drug companies for further investigating the value of these drugs for cancer treatment.

WHY OFF-LABEL USE?

Why are drugs used for indications other than those they were designed for? The answer is simple. Although drugs usually affect the human body in many different ways, the FDA routinely approves them for just a single use or action. For example: aspirin for headaches, diphenhydramine (Benedryl) for allergies, and propranolol (Inderal) to control high blood pressure and heart rhythm. Yet over time, other beneficial effects are discovered. Thus, aspirin is also commonly used as a blood thinner, Benedryl as a sleeping pill, and propranolol as an anti-anxiety medication. In fact, many drugs work better and become much more successful in their off-label use than for their primary purpose.

In many cases, an off-label use was established by reports from people who took these medications for one condition and noticed that another one improved. For example, people taking propranolol for high blood pressure discovered that their anxiety had subsided. Many such anecdotal reports enabled physicians to define these off-label uses. Often off-label uses were actually discovered by the pharmaceutical companies that develped these drugs. So why should off-label use of medications for treating cancer be any different?

In fact, though less widespread, off-label drugs are successful as weapons against cancer. I've written this chapter in case one or more of these drugs may be able to help you or someone you love to survive. Perhaps you already know someone they've helped. Maybe that someone is you.

Here are the off-label drugs that I and most other integrative cancer specialists find most useful:

- Low-dose naltrexone (LDN)
- Metformin (Glucophage)
- Cimetidine (Tagamet)
- Celecoxib (Celebrex)
- Statins
- Ammonium tetrathiomolybdate (ATTM)

- Dichloroacetic acid (DCA)
- Doxycycline
- Amiloride
- Dipyrimadole (Persantine)
- Disulfiram (Antabuse)
- Nelfinavir (Viracept)
- Methazolamide

These drugs are not used as stand-alone treatments for cancer. They're prescribed as part of an entire integrative program.

LOW-DOSE NALTREXONE—A WELL-KEPT SECRET

Integrative physicians generally agree that low-dose naltrexone (LDN) may be one of the best-kept secrets of the last thirty years: a safe, inexpensive treatment that stimulates a person's immune system. Naltrexone was originally approved by the FDA in 1984 in a dose of 50 mg to treat heroin or opium addiction. The drug blocks the experience of euphoria that these opioid (narcotic) drugs produce by preventing opioid receptors on cell membranes from taking them in.

In 1985 Bernard Bihari, M.D., a New York physician, discovered that a much smaller dose of naltrexone, 3–4.5 mg per day taken at bedtime, could boost the immune system response of patients with HIV/AIDS. During the 1990s, he noticed that low doses of naltrexone also helped patients with different types of cancer, including lymphoma and pancreatic cancer, as well as those with autoimmune diseases like systemic lupus erythematosis (SLE). He and other physicians later reported that

LDN also benefited people with a variety of other disorders, including amyotrophic lateral sclerosis (ALS—Lou Gehrig's disease), ankylosing spondylitis, Crohn's disease, chronic obstructive pulmonary disease (COPD), Hashimoto's thyroiditis, multiple sclerosis, Parkinson's, psoriasis, rheumatoid arthritis, and a long list of cancers (Jill in Chapter 4 took LDN as part of a treatment program for breast cancer).

How LDN Works

In addition to blocking the opioids in drugs, LDN blocks the natural opioid hormones produced by the brain and adrenal glands: endorphins and enkephalins. People with cancer and other diseases tend to be deficient in these hormones. It may sound contradictory, but this blocking effect actually helps restore the body's normal level of endorphin and enkephalin production.

Almost every cell in the body has receptors for these hormones, including immune system cells. Over the last two decades, much evidence has accumulated indicating that these internal opioids play a significant role in immune-system modulation. These natural opioids act like cytokines, stimulating the immune system by way of the opioid receptors on the immune cells. It seems that taking LDN at bedtime causes blocking of opioid receptors in the middle of the night, which stimulates increased production of endorphin and enkephalin. These hormones then act as immune system boosters.

LDN's immune-enhancing ability has found multiple medical applications. In 1994, a researcher first noted that the recent (at that time) discovery that immune cells had receptors for opioids probably meant that opioids directly affected the immune system.[1] By 2003, an article in the *New England Journal of Medicine* referred to extensive evidence that opioids affect "the development, differentiation, and function of immune cells,"[2] including macrophages, natural killer cells, T cells, and B cells—major soldiers of the immune system. In laboratory studies, endorphins and LDN inhibited a number of different human tumors. Researchers hypothesize that the increased endorphin and enkephalin levels produced by LDN activate the tumor's opioid receptors, which induces apoptosis of the tumor cells. A second mechanism of LDN's action is to increase the number of natural killer cells and other immune defenses against cancer.

Given these facts, it's clear that LDN successfully addresses the immune connection.

LDN and Cancer

In 2004, Dr. Bihari reported the results of treating over 300 of his patients whose cancers did not respond to the conventional trio. After four to six months of taking LDN, half of them showed signs that their tumors had stopped growing. And a third showed objective signs that their tumors had actually shrunk.

Researchers have found opioid receptors in brain tumors, breast cancers, endometrial cancers, head and neck cancers, squamous cell carcinoma, myeloid leukemia, both small cell and non-small-cell lung cancer, neuroblastoma, and others, which means that all these cancers are prospects for treatment with LDN. (*See below* for the list of cancers that Dr. Bihari and others have found responsive to LDN.)

Cancers Responsive to LDN

LDN is taken as a pill at bedtime in a dose of 4.5 mg.

- Bladder cancer
- Breast cancer
- Carcinoid
- Colon and rectal cancer
- Glioblastoma
- Liver cancer
- Lung cancer (non-small cell)
- Lymphocytic leukemia (chronic)
- Lymphoma (Hodgkin's and non-Hodgkin's)
- Malignant melanoma
- Multiple myeloma
- Neuroblastoma
- Ovarian cancer
- Pancreatic cancer
- Prostate cancer (untreated)
- Renal cell carcinoma
- Throat cancer
- Uterine cancer

METFORMIN AND THE CANCER CONNECTIONS

Metformin was designed to treat type 2 (non-insulin-dependent) diabetes. Derived from a substance found in a plant called goat's rue or
French lilac (*Gallega officinalis*), it is one of the safest, most commonly
prescribed medications for diabetes. Like insulin, metformin works by
decreasing the level of glucose in the blood, thus removing the only food
that cancer cells find palatable. Metformin lowers blood sugar through
the following mechanisms.

- It suppresses hepatic gluconeogenesis (production of sugar by the liver).

- It increases insulin sensitivity.

- It enhances the body's utilization of sugar.

- It decreases absorption of sugar in the intestine (meaning that less
  sugar enters the bloodstream).

The result is an improvement in overall sugar metabolism, since the
smaller amount of sugar present is metabolized very quickly. In fact, metformin has several off-label uses for conditions that involve faulty sugar
metabolism, including polycystic ovary syndrome (PCOS), infertility,
syndrome X (metabolic syndrome), and nonalcoholic fatty liver disease.
So you won't be surprised to hear that, like IPT-LD (*see* Chapter 4), metformin is also an excellent weapon against cancer.

Lab studies, animal studies, and some clinical evidence support metformin's use for cancer treatment. Researchers have observed several
mechanisms by which it causes apoptosis in cancer cells, pointing to a
genetic connection. It prevented pancreatic cancer in hamsters, inhibited
development of breast cancer in mice, and suppressed growth of precancerous intestinal polyps and growth of lung cancer in mice. Metformin
also inhibited the growth of prostate cancer cells and reduced tumor
growth in mice.[3]

Even more exciting are results from clinical studies of patients who
took metformin. A team of Scottish researchers who reviewed ten years of
patient records concluded that those who had taken metformin for type 2
diabetes had a reduced risk of cancer.[4] A research team at the MD Anderson Cancer Center studied 155 test subjects with diabetes among a total

of 2,529 women receiving neoadjuvant chemotherapy for early-stage breast cancer. Of these 155, the 87 who were taking metformin had a pathologic complete response rate (a complete disappearance of cancer cells) of 24 percent, three times higher than the rate of 8 percent among the 68 women who were not taking metformin. The rate among the women who did not have diabetes was 16 percent. These results are pretty convincing, and not just to me, but also to the researchers, who planned a further study combining metformin with hormone therapy to treat obese women with metastatic breast cancer (metformin is also known to help battle obesity).

I became particularly enthusiastic about metformin when I learned personally from the late Professor Dilman that he had successfully used phenformin, an earlier version of the drug, to treat breast cancer and endometrial cancer in experiments conducted in the 1960s and 1970s. Dilman also treated MID successfully with phenformin. If you add all these up—sugar, genetic, obesity, and MID, you see that metformin addresses four of the cancer connections. I use metformin for almost every cancer patient, especially those with breast, prostate, and colon cancer.

Doses of metformin range from 500 mg twice a day to 1,000 mg twice a day, depending on the person's blood sugar and hemoglobin A1c levels. (Hemoglobin A1c is an indicator of how well blood sugar was controlled over the previous three months.)

CIMETIDINE: ANOTHER CANCER BUSTER

Cimetidine (Tagamet) has been known as a stomach-acid inhibitor since the 1970s. This over-the-counter drug is commonly taken for peptic ulcers and heartburn. It's also used off-label to treat fibromyalgia, HIV, hives, irritable bowel syndrome, shingles, and warts, as well as for weight control, among other uses.

As an anti-cancer drug, cimetidine hits the jackpot. Its anti-tumor effects were first noticed in 1979 in a report of two cancer cases in *The Lancet*. The first was a man with metastasized head and neck cancer who had refused chemotherapy. He was taking cimetidine for an upset stomach, and lo and behold, his metastases disappeared. The second case was a woman with lung cancer that had metastasized to her brain.

She happened to use cimetidine for heartburn, and her tumors shrank.[5]

Subsequent test-tube studies, animal research, and clinical research provided evidence that cimetidine has immune-boosting effects, as well as anti-tumor effects in melanomas and in cancers of the colon, esophagus, gallbladder, kidney, liver, ovary, and stomach. For example, Australian researchers compared treatment for metastatic colon cancer with chemo and cimetidine combined, and with chemo alone. They found a 36 percent improvement in the CEA tumor marker in the chemo-plus-cimetidine group and no improvement in the chemo-only group. Japanese and Danish researchers both reported that adding cimetidine to a chemo regimen for people with colon and colorectal cancer increased survival. The ones in the groups that took cimetidine had a median survival rate of four years, in comparison to a median survival rate of only two years among the groups who didn't take it. The best results were for rectal cancer; all those taking cimetidine survived four years, compared to half of the control group. In cases of renal cell carcinoma, which is particularly tough to treat, researchers who used a combination of cimetidine and interferon reported some positive response.[6]

Cimetidine's mechanisms of action are explained as follows:

- It inhibits the adhesive quality of tumor cells, which they require for metastasis.

- Histamine is a growth factor for certain types of tumor cells, and cimetidine blocks the action of histamines and their receptors on cell membranes.

- It boosts the immune system by inhibiting T cell suppressor activity.

- It inhibits angiogenesis. (I mention this effect of cimetidine because the question is still unresolved.)

- It stimulates production of the cytokine interleukin-2.

An anti-cancer dose of cimetidine is 1,200–1,600 mg per day. However, it must be prescribed by a doctor for treating cancer because it has many possible drug interactions. I like to use cimetidine as part of treatment for colon cancer.

CELECOXIB: A CANCER TERMINATOR

Celecoxib (Celebrex), a popular arthritis-buster whose anti-inflammatory properties relieve pain, swelling, and tenderness, can also terminate many cancers. It has two different anti-cancer actions.

First, a research group at Winship Cancer Institute of Emory University found that this drug has a smart-bomb effect: it activates a "death" receptor that causes cancer cells to self destruct.[7] The Winship researchers' work confirmed previous reports that celecoxib fights cancer quite differently from the way it fights arthritis. Their fascinating discovery was that celecoxib intrudes into a molecular keyhole receptor on the outer surface of the cancer cell (the death receptor). The FDA has already approved celecoxib to treat adenomatous polyposis (development of polyps), a precursor to colon cancer.

Second, celecoxib's anti-inflammatory properties reduce the risk of developing these precancerous colon polyps in the first place. Celecoxib is a COX-2 inhibitor that blocks the COX-2 enzyme, a major cause of inflammation. It's known to be beneficial not only for colorectal cancer, but also for lung cancer caused by smoking. I'm sure you've already figured out that this is the inflammation connection. And celecoxib absolutely addresses it.

However, celecoxib does present two problems. First, it poses an increased risk of heart attack. Some physicians believe this is because it prevents angiogenesis and therefore limits the supply of oxygen to the heart. Thus many with cancer have to make a tough choice—to help their cancer or hurt their heart. If their cancer is far advanced, though, they don't really have much choice—they need to take the celecoxib and take the risk, just as often happens with the chemo drug Adriamycin, which also causes heart problems.

This brings up the second problem. Because of the risk of heart attack, many cancer patients in the original research trials stopped taking celecoxib. Then, during their follow-up visits after the trials were completed, it turned out that 27 percent had developed new polyps (rather like a rebound effect), compared with 16 percent who had taken a placebo. Thus those who took celecoxib had a 66 percent higher risk of developing new polyps.[8]

I myself use celecoxib as part of an integrative program for patients with colorectal cancer. Whether or not to take it is, of course, decided individually in each case.

The recommended dose of celecoxib for cancer treatment is 400 mg twice a day.

STATINS—NOT JUST FOR HIGH CHOLESTEROL

Statins, the second most commonly prescribed group of drugs (after analgesics), are well known for lowering high cholesterol. They work by blocking the enzyme HMG-CoA reductase, which the liver needs to manufacture cholesterol. But statins have a diverse array of other actions that have led to a number of off-label uses: they help treat autoimmune problems, cancer, cataracts, COPD, osteoporosis, and PCOS, among other conditions.

Statins' anti-inflammatory, immunomodulatory, and anti-angiogenic properties are responsible for their anti-cancer effects. And since their cholesterol-lowering actions effectively reverse MID, adding up these activities shows that statins address the immune, inflammation, and MID connections.

Different statins work better against different cancers, depending on whether the drugs are lipophilic (fat soluble, like simvastatin, or Zocor) or hydrophilic (water soluble, like pravastatin, or Pravachol). Evidence from lab studies on cancer cells indicates that statins are helpful for brain, breast, colon, lung, ovarian, pancreatic, and prostate cancers. Animal studies reveal statins to have powerful preventive and suppressive anti-cancer effects. Most clinical trials have tested either statins' ability to prevent cancer or their value as an adjuvant treatment. Positive results were reported in cases of breast, colorectal, lung, and prostate cancer, and in hepatocarcinoma.[9]

Statins are quite user-friendly. They work synergistically with chemo drugs (cisplatin, doxorubicin, Gemzar, herceptin, Nexavar, Taxol, and others). Statins also work well in conjunction with other off-label drugs (celecoxib and other non-steroidal anti-inflammatory drugs—NSAIDs) and with natural substances (all-trans retinoic acid or ATRA, gamma tocotrienols, and green tea polyphenols).

The major concern with statins is that they suppress liver function, which is why some physicians no longer use them to lower cholesterol. They have other, less serious, side effects as well. So when statins are prescribed, the patient's liver function is monitored. Most do well, but a few need to stop taking the drug. There are so many statins that there's no point in specifying doses here; in any case, the dosage is the same as for treating high cholesterol.

AMMONIUM TETRATHIOMOLYBDATE

More conveniently referred to as ATTM, ammonium tetrathiomolybdate is known as a treatment for Wilson's disease, a hereditary disorder in which excess copper builds up in tissues. ATTM works by preventing tissues from absorbing copper and by increasing its excretion. That's where its value for treating cancer comes in. Tumors need copper to turn on the process of angiogenesis, so by removing copper from the body, it seems, ATTM can prevent angiogenesis.

Nevertheless, a question remains in my mind about the assumption underlying this treatment. Most integrative physicians use ATTM because they want to inhibit angiogenesis. As you know, I believe that preventing angiogenesis is not necessarily beneficial. Inhibiting angiogenesis means cutting the oxygen supply to the tumor, which, as Chapter 6 explained, may actually stimulate cancer growth. Theoretically, my concern about preventing angiogenesis is quite justified, but many experts still maintain that doing so is beneficial.

It will take many years and much research to resolve the angiogenesis controversy. Two things are certain, however: an elevated copper level is essential for angiogenesis to happen, and ATTM can lower copper levels. And since I suspect that preventing angiogenesis may not be desirable, until the question is settled, I don't use ATTM.

DICHLOROACETIC ACID

Dichloroacetic acid (DCA) is a byproduct of the chlorination of drinking water. The pure chemical is a strong acid that can burn tissues. Sodium dichloroacetate is the form that is used as a medication.

Laboratory studies indicate that DCA inhibits glycolysis and restores the action of the mitochondria in cancer cells, helping oxidate them. As you know, cancer cells rely heavily on sugar intake and much prefer oxygen-deprived mitochondria that can't function well. Interruption of their sugar supply and greater mitochondrial efficiency are exactly what cancer cells *don't* want to experience. And that's precisely what DCA does. In 2009, researchers at Medicor Cancer Centers in Canada reported the results of treating 179 people who had cancer with DCA. Sixty percent had a positive response. Of these, 12 percent had reduced tumor size, 9 percent had a reduction in tumor markers, 7 percent showed improvement in their blood tests, and in 34 percent their disease stabilized.[10]

Doses are 20–25 mg/kg per day for adults and 25–50 mg/kg per day for children. DCA is taken for two weeks, followed by a one-week break. This cycle is then repeated as directed by the physician.

DCA has side effects that may be annoying, but are transient and not serious. They include fatigue, numbness, tremor, and loss of balance.

DOXYCYCLINE

It turns out that doxycycline, an antibiotic long used to treat various infections, can also inhibit the growth of different types of cancer cells as well as induce apoptosis. One of its actions is to prevent cancer cells from releasing the enzyme metalloproteinase (MMP), which degrades and dismantles tissues, paving the way for cancer metastasis. In cell research, doxycycline inhibited the growth of prostate cancer cells and shrank the tumor size of bone metastases of breast cancer. It inhibited non-small-cell lung cancer cell lines and induced apoptosis in pancreatic cancer and glioblastoma cells. Doxycycline also inhibits the chemical process by which melanoma cells become adhesive, or sticky, a mechanism that enables them to metastasize. These same cells then undergo apoptosis.[11]

Doxycycline is taken orally in a dose of 200 mg per day for several months.

AMILORIDE

Amiloride is a well-known diuretic that promotes excretion of salt and water in the urine, without excess loss of potassium. It's used mainly to treat congestive heart failure and hypertension, usually in combination with other diuretics.

Amiloride also has anti-cancer effects. Chinese researchers have found that it can inhibit several cancer cell lines by changing the instructions cancer-cell genes transmit in order to make new proteins. Abnormal instructions are associated with malignant cells that are invasive and able to resist chemotherapy. The researchers found that treating such cells with amiloride disrupted their ability to reproduce and invade other tissues. These changes led to apoptosis.[12]

Another anti-cancer effect of amiloride has to do with its ability to lower sodium levels. Cancer-cell nuclei have a higher sodium level than do the nuclei of normal cells. Researchers at the University of Texas Health Science Center, speculating that this high sodium might play a role in cancer development, injected amiloride into mice that had a type of liver cancer. They found that the drug both inhibited tumor growth and decreased cancer-cell proliferation. These changes were associated with lower sodium within cell nuclei, suggesting that the drug's effect had to do with the decreased sodium level.[13]

The dose of amiloride is 5–10 mg twice a day, as tolerated, for several weeks. Integrative physicians have begun using amiloride relatively recently, but as of this writing, I myself have not yet used it.

DIPYRIMADOLE (PERSANTINE)

Dipyrimadole is an older drug used with or without aspirin to lower the risk of blood clots in order to prevent strokes and heart attacks. Researchers have studied its possible uses against cancer for quite a while, and in fact the National Cancer Institute website notes that dipyrimadole enhances the effectiveness of chemotherapy. In cell studies, it enhanced the cytotoxic effects of Adriamycin, cisplatin, etoposide, 5-FU, interferon, methotrexate, and vinblastin.[14]

In 1987, the results of a large European study on preventing strokes were published. Test subjects who'd had a stroke were given either dipyrimadole plus aspirin or placebo. Those who got the dipyrimadole had a 30 percent reduction in cancer mortality.[15] The researchers speculated that the drug prevented tumor cells from attaching to the lining of blood vessels (which is, in fact, one of the actions of this type of drug, known as an antithrombotic).

You might conclude that this action of dipyrimadole could be useful as a cancer-treatment strategy. And you'd be right. In fact, the idea that antithrombotic drugs have an anti-cancer effect was initially proposed in 1958. In 1964, a report noted that coumadin (another antithrombotic agent) could reduce mortality from lung cancer. The same anti-cancer effect was reported in cell studies of other thrombolytic drugs—aspirin, heparin, and hydroxychloroquine. In animal studies, dipyrimadole prevented development of metastases in mice with pancreatic cancer. And in clinical studies, dipyrimadole was beneficial in treating melanoma and gastric and pancreatic cancer.[16] These results reinforce the importance of the thrombolytic effect for anti-cancer activity.

The dose is the same as for standard treatment uses.

DISULFIRAM (ANTABUSE)

Disulfiram has a long history as a treatment for alcoholism and cocaine addiction. There are also numerous reports of disulfiram's cancer-inhibiting properties. Since the 1970s, multiple cell and animal studies have demonstrated that it can reduce resistance to chemo drugs, reduce the invasiveness of tumor cells, and inhibit a genetic mechanism needed for angiogenesis.[17]

There is also one clinical report that disulfiram taken with zinc gluconate resulted in more than 50 percent reduction in liver metastases and clinical remission in a patient with stage-4 metastatic melanoma of the eye. The person continued on this medication for over four years with very few side effects.[18]

The initial dose of disulfiram is 500 mg per day for one to two weeks, followed by a maintenance dose of 250 mg per day for several weeks.

NELFINAVIR (VIRACEPT)

Nelfinavir is a protease inhibitor that prevents the HIV virus from replicating itself. Apart from its use to treat HIV/AIDS, it can also prevent cancer cells from spreading. Researchers at the National Cancer Institute Center for Cancer Research took six existing HIV protease inhibitors and tested them against nine different types of cancer cells. They found that nelfinavir had the most potent anti-cancer activity. It prevented tumor growth and induced cell death both through apoptosis and through autophagy, a process of self-digestion that occurs when the cell is under stress.[19] Nelfinavir also showed immune-modulating properties and anti-angiogenic activity.

Other researchers found that nelfinavir made cancer cells more sensitive to radiation.[20] One small trial in which patients with advanced pancreatic cancer were treated with nelfinavir plus the conventional duo resulted in dramatic improvement in six out of ten patients.[21] In 2011, the National Cancer Institute was conducting phase 1 and 2 studies to evaluate nelfinavir's activity against a range of different cancers, by itself and together with the conventional duo and other drugs.

The usual dose of nelfinavir is 1,250 mg twice a day for several weeks. As of this writing, I have not yet used it.

METHAZOLAMIDE

Methazolamide is usually used to treat glaucoma. But it's also been found to improve the oxygenation of solid tumors, which means it may be able to make radiation therapy more effective. Solid tumors are often hard to treat with radiation and chemo, and scientists suspect this is because cancer cells are low in oxygen. The best way to oxygenate cells, as I explained in the previous chapter, is to use oxygen therapies. An alternate method would be to give methazolamide.

Since about two-thirds of women with cervical cancer receive radiation as part of their treatment, testing whether methazolamide can improve their response to therapy would be extremely helpful. In fact, a clinical trial of methazolamide for cervical cancer was planned, but had to be withdrawn for lack of funds. (At this point, I'm getting so tired of having to say that such-and-such method was not researched for lack of funding that I sometimes ponder changing my vocation from physician to financier.)

Despite this lack of research, I include methazolamide here because it's part of the oral medication regimen in the protocol developed by Mark Rosenberg, M.D., which the next section describes.

DR. ROSENBERG'S CANCER PH
MANIPULATION THERAPY

Mark Rosenberg, M.D., is director of the Fellowship in Integrative Cancer Therapy of the American Academy of Anti-Aging Medicine— the program described in the preface that I myself graduated from. Dr. Rosenberg is a charismatic, energetic, ambitious physician and researcher who has developed a new anti-cancer modality he calls Cancer pH Manipulation Therapy. Using this protocol, in just four weeks, and without any conventional therapy, he completely normalized tumor markers in a patient of his with metastatic endometrial carcinoma. For a second patient, he reduced tumor markers by 40 percent in only two weeks. And this brand-new treatment is only in its early stage.

What's the rationale behind his treatment? You already know about the connection between pH and cancer. Rosenberg goes much deeper into it than anyone else. His protocol consists of the following.

- Oral administration of eight different drugs, based on their off-label therapeutic properties—amiloride, ATTM, celecoxib, cimetidine, esomeprazole (Nexium), hydrochlorothiazide (HCTZ), metformin, and methazolamide.

- A high-dose IV infusion of glucose, together with slow insulin drip.

- A high dose of probiotics every day, plus pancreatic enzymes.

This regimen sounds rather gruesome—and more seriously, it may seem to contradict much of what I've been saying up to this point. But let me analyze it carefully based on the idea that a major principle in preventing cancer and metastasis is keeping the pH alkaline.

Here's why Rosenberg infuses lots of glucose into the cancer-affected body. In the advanced stages of cancer, cancer cells are full of lactic acid, and therefore extremely acidic. This lactic acid travels across the cancer-cell membrane, from the interior of the cell into the space between cells (the intercellular space) and back again. But if a way can be found to close the gate in the cell membrane to prevent the lactic acid from getting out—essentially incarcerate it inside the cell, while also pumping more lactic acid into the cell to increase its acidity—the extreme acidity that builds up will at length corrode the cell and burn it out, and it will die. Most important of all, the stem cells, which as you may recall, are untouchable by chemotherapy in advanced cancer, are vulnerable to this acidity. So they are killed as well.

How then to keep that lactic acid locked inside the cancer cell? That's the job of the off-label drugs—they block the outflow of lactic acid from the cell, and, as I've explained, when acidity can leak out of the cell into the intercellular space, apoptosis will not happen. So, you see, the pH connection is quite complex. You want the intercellular space to be alkaline, but you want the interior of the cancer cell to be very acidic. The acidity inside the cancer cell will kill it, while the alkaline intercellular space enables normal cells to undergo apoptosis, thus preventing them from becoming cancerous. When the intercellular space is acidic, apoptosis will not take place; that's how cancer cells remain immortal.

Rosenberg's eight-drug combination is given for several weeks. Then, once the outflow of lactic acid from the cells is blocked, the glucose IV infusion is administered to increase the lactic acid inside the cells. Locked up behind the cell membrane, this additional lactic acid can't escape. The IV glucose plus insulin is given once a week until the treatment is complete (according to his patient's response). Good luck to you, Dr. Rosenberg, in your further research.

FINAL THOUGHTS

While I was thinking about this chapter, the U.S. Postal Service slogan "If it fits, it ships!" popped into my mind. So simple, so clear. Everything that fits into their box or envelope will be shipped wherever you want to send it. When it comes to cancer therapies, though, not everything that fits (makes sense) will be shipped (used as a treatment).

So why is off-label use of drugs such a good fit as part of an overall integrative treatment program? You'll say it's because they address many of the cancer connections—and you could not be more right.

- DCA, metformin, and statins address the genetic, MID, obesity, and sugar connections.

- Cimetidine, LDN, nelfinavir, and statins address the immune connection.

- Celebrex and statins address the inflammation connection.

- Celecoxib, doxycycline, metformin, and nelfinavir address the genetic connection.

- All the drugs in Rosenberg's protocol address the pH connection.

- Methazolamide addresses the oxygen connection.

Even though these off-label uses are so simple, their value so obvious, and the drugs so easily available, I need to once again point out that integrative cancer physicians are the only doctors using them—at least for now.

CHAPTER 8

- - - - -

Natural Substances
Fight Cancer with a Vengeance

INITIAL THOUGHTS

As I sat down to write this chapter, I said to myself, "I'm in trouble!" Such a huge number of natural cancer remedies have been reported in the literature that I initially wasn't sure which ones to describe and how much to say about them. There are whole books devoted just to a single natural substance. Other books spend an entire chapter on one supplement. So it was quite a challenge to figure out how to discuss all the supplements that treat cancer in one chapter. But I soon hit upon the most sensible, logical arrangement. This chapter describes natural substances according to how they address the different cancer connections. That makes sense to me, and I trust it does to you as well.

Chapter 2 described natural substances that relieve, or ward off, the toxic side effects of the conventional trio and may in addition improve the efficacy of these treatments. That chapter also discussed combining antioxidants with the conventional trio. I strongly suggest you revisit Chapter 2 before reading this one, which presents natural substances that fight cancer directly. An unlimited number of reports describe how such substances have helped people with advanced cancer survive the unsurvivable. *Most important, these substances only kill the cancer cells, not the people themselves.* I've never heard of anyone with cancer who is scared of taking nutritional supplements the way they're scared of chemo. In fact, most people walk into an integrative physician's office toting bags full of the various supplements they've already included in their treatment protocols.

For various reasons, many of my readers won't be getting treatment from an integrative oncologist. But if they can at least use the information in this chapter to help themselves survive their cancers, my mission will be accomplished.

There are three points to keep in mind.

- When I give a range of dosages for a substance, always begin with the lowest dose. Then, if you tolerate the remedy well, move to a higher dose.

- Quite a few of the natural substances described below address more than one cancer connection, and some are listed more than once.

- Many supplements described here have anti-angiogenic properties. I have included them because I haven't yet decided whether preventing angiogenesis is beneficial or not. At this point, I suggest you take them for two reasons. First, they have many other anti-cancer properties. Second, I don't want to tell you not to take them because no one yet knows the answer to the anti-angiogenesis dilemma. Much research must be done to find it, and I'm sure more than a decade will be needed to come to a definite conclusion.

THE GENETIC CONNECTION— NATURAL SUBSTANCES WITH CYTOTOXIC EFFECTS

A number of nutritional substances have cytotoxic properties and thus can act as natural chemo agents. They do this primarily by addressing the genetic connection, through the following general mechanisms.

- Blocking key physiological processes (known as signal transduction pathways) required for cancer-cell replication.

- Triggering the pathway that induces cancer-cell apoptosis.

- Enhancing detoxification processes that neutralize and eliminate carcinogens in the body.

- Blocking the synthesis of dangerous types of estrogen and testosterone associated with breast, ovarian, and prostate cancer.

- Promoting better cell differentiation, thereby decreasing the risk that healthy cells will turn into cancerous ones.

- Blocking receptor sites on cells to prevent overstimulation of growth factors and hormones, thereby slowing down the rate of cell division.

- Slowing down the rate of cell replication, thus reducing the frequency of genetic mutations.

Graviola (*Annona Muricata*)

Also known as soursop or guanabana, graviola is an evergreen tree native to the tropics. It is remarkably cytotoxic to cancer cells, but not to healthy cells. Researchers at Purdue University found that compounds in the bark of the tree can fight some cancers that are drug resistant. One compound, called bullatacin, inhibited ATP production, thereby eliminating the cancer's energy source.[1]

Powdered graviola is available in capsules. Follow the dosages on the bottle.

Poly-MVA

Poly-MVA is a patented dietary supplement whose main ingredients are the mineral palladium bonded with alpha-lipoic acid, vitamins, minerals, and amino acids. According to research conducted at the Garnett McKeen Laboratory, Poly-MVA helps healthy cells produce energy, supports liver detoxification, helps prevent cell damage by radiation, and enhances white blood cell function.[2]

The recommended dose is two teaspoons four times a day, thirty minutes before meals and before bedtime for the first two months. Then take two teaspoons twice a day, thirty minutes before meals.

Essential Fatty Acids (EFAs)

The EFAs with the greatest anti-cancer activity are eicosapentaenoic acid (EPA) and docosahexaenoic acid (DHA). These are omega-3 fatty acids that come from wild, deep-sea sourced fish oils. EFAs can:

- Reduce production of the inflammation-promoting enzyme COX-2;

- Reduce vascular endothelial growth factor (VEGF), thus preventing angiogenesis;

- Make some chemo drugs more effective;

- Reduce tumor growth;

- Suppress a cancer-growth-promoting protein known as Bas.

I use my own supplement, Super Omega Guard. Two capsules contain 900 mg of EPA, 660 mg of DHA, and 1,000 IU of vitamin D_3 (cholecalciferol). I recommend two capsules twice a day. Look for a product that gives you approximately the same levels of supplements.

Vitamin D

Vitamin D has numerous anti-cancer activities. Researchers have suggested several mechanisms to explain how it works. Among other actions, vitamin D:

- Is associated with high levels of a molecule that prevents epithelial cells from becoming malignant;

- Stabilizes the cell cycle, preventing out-of-control cell growth;

- Promotes apoptosis;

- Prevents new angiogenesis.

The best form to use as a supplement is vitamin D_3. Dosage is 7,000–10,000 IU per day.

Be sure to ask your physician to do a 25-hydroxy vitamin-D test, to check your blood level of vitamin D_3. In cancer patients, the range should be 60–90 nanograms per milliliter (ng/mL). If the number is below 60, take the higher dosage. The idea is to adjust the dosage to keep your vitamin D_3 level within this range.

Cruciferous Vegetable Extracts

Cruciferous vegetables, such as broccoli and cabbage, are rich in sulfur-containing compounds known as isothiocyanates. Two isothiocyanates, benzyl isothiocyanate (BITC) and sulforaphane, have been widely reported to have anti-cancer properties, although exactly how they work is not yet fully understood. What is known is:

- BITC induces apoptosis in some types of pancreatic cancer cells;

- Sulforaphane, the most studied isothiocyanate, blocks the growth phases of the cell cycle of chemically induced tumors in animals;

- Sulforaphane increases the efficacy of doxyrubicin in mice;

- Sulforaphane has anti-metastatic activity;

- Sulforaphane inhibits the progression of lung adenomas.

I use my proprietary formula, Onco Guard, which contains a patented form of sulforaphane called BroccoRaphanin. Each capsule contains 500 mg, and the suggested dose is one capsule three times a day. You can buy any product containing sulforaphane.

Resveratrol

Resveratrol is a compound found in the skin of red grapes. In 2008, researchers at the University of Rochester Medical Center reported that, when taken in high doses, it acts as a pro-oxidant (just like high doses of vitamin C—*see* Chapter 3) and kills cancer cells, without harming healthy cells.[3]

Resveratrol also:

- Makes radiation therapy more effective;

- Inhibits production of matrix metalloproteinase 2, an enzyme used by cancer cells to break down cell membranes so they can metastasize;

- Induces apoptosis.

Resveratrol is effective for treating breast, colon, esophageal, prostate, and skin cancers. It can be used in all three stages of cancer development—initiation, promotion, and progression.

Recommended dosage: 2,000 mg per day, divided into two doses.

Curcumin

Curcumin is one of several compounds called curcuminoids that give the Indian curry spice turmeric (*Curcuma longa*) its yellow color. A Korean study concluded that it has a powerful ability to both prevent and treat cancer.[4] Curcumin:

- Is an antioxidant;

- Inhibits angiogenesis;

- Prevents tumor cells from invading normal tissue;

- Induces apoptosis;

- Prevents breast stem cells from reproducing, yet is not toxic to regular differentiated cells, suggesting that turmeric can be a potent cancer-preventive agent.

  Dosage: Two 875-mg capsules per day.

Tea

Yes, ordinary tea that you may already drink every day. Both black and green tea have multiple anti-cancer effects. However, for cancer-fighting purposes, green tea is preferable. It has been more extensively studied, so more about its benefits is known. The active anti-cancer components in green tea leaves are four polyphenols (antioxidant compounds found in plants): epigallocatechin gallate (EGCG), epigallocatechin, epicatechin gallate (ECG), and epicatechin.

- According to a joint U.S. Department of Agriculture/South Korean team of researchers, most of the polyphenols in green and black tea that were studied decreased a number of cancer-cell lines, including human breast, liver (hepatoma), and prostate cancer cells.[5]

- Different studies have suggested that tea flavonoids (a flavonoid is a type of polyphenol) can induce apoptosis; stop P-450 enzymes, which activate carcinogens; block transmission of signals by cancer promoters; bind to damaged DNA involved in cancer promotion; and inhibit angiogenesis.

- Mayo Clinic researchers reported that EGCG halted disease progression in the majority of forty-two patients with early-stage chronic lymphocytic leukemia.[6]

- In an epidemiological study, an ECG blood level of 9.3 ng/ml or greater corresponded to a 75 percent reduction in the risk of gastric cancer. That is, people who drank more black or green tea had a lower risk for this type of cancer.

- In other studies, a reduced incidence and severity of lung, stomach, colon, pancreatic, liver, breast, prostate, and skin cancers was associated with green tea consumption.

- Still another study found that both smokers and nonsmokers who drank green tea had over five times less risk of lung cancer. A study of lung cancer came up with the same result.

To attain the necessary blood level of polyphenols for an anti-cancer effect, you need to drink at least eight cups of green tea a day. More conveniently, you can buy capsules or tablets of green tea extract. The suggested dose is 2,000 mg of green tea extract per day.

Selenium

Supplementation with the trace mineral selenium leads to increased levels of methylated selenium, a metabolite of selenium (a product resulting from metabolizing it) that is mainly responsible for selenium's cancer-preventive effects.

- Apoptosis usually occurs when the plasma-selenium concentration is approximately 120–200 micromol/liter.

- Selenium inhibits cancer cell growth.

- It activates the P53 tumor-suppressor gene.

- It protects against DNA damage.

- It disrupts cancer cell division.

- At blood levels of 120 micromol/liter, it reduces the risk of colon cancer by 50 percent or more.

Recommended dosage: 200–400 mcg of selenium per day.

In my opinion, selenium and vitamin D are the key supplements for treating prostate cancer.

Quercetin

Found in fruits and many other plants, quercetin is one of the most effective anti-cancer flavonoids. Its mechanisms of action include the following:

- Inhibition of tyrosine kinase, an enzyme that plays an important role in the process by which cells become malignant;

- Inhibition of lipoxygenase (LOX), an enzyme involved in the inflammatory process;

- Enhancing the efficacy of chemotherapy while decreasing its side effects;

- Inhibition of angiogenesis;

  Recommended dosage: 500–1,000 mg, three times a day.

Feverfew

Parthenolide, the active ingredient of the feverfew plant (*Tanacetum parthenium*), has several anti-cancer properties.

- It's a potent inhibitor of DNA synthesis and cell proliferation in many human cancers.

- It has well-documented anti-inflammatory properties (the inflammation connection).

- In cell studies, parthenolide induced apoptosis by activating an enzyme called caspase-3.

- In other cell studies, parthenolide destroyed acute myeloid leukemia (AML) cells.

  The suggested dosage is 4 mg per day.

Milk Thistle

Milk thistle (*Silybum marianum*) contains a flavonoid called silymarin, whose main active component is silibinin. Silibinin and the other flavonoids in milk thistle may benefit a number of disorders, including alcoholic cirrhosis (a precancerous condition) and tumors. In particular, these compounds have shown extremely potent anti-prostate-cancer and anti-lung-cancer activity.

- Silibinin modifies the cell cycle, inhibiting cancer cell growth, and also activates caspase-3, causing apoptosis. One study found a strong indication that silibinim has a cytotoxic effect on bladder cancer cells.[7]

  Recommended dosage: 200–800 mg per day.

CoEnzyme Q$_{10}$

The great majority of cancer patients have low CoQ$_{10}$ levels, and it's well worth taking this supplement to raise the level. In Chapter 2, I described the benefits of CoQ$_{10}$ when used together with the conventional treatment trio. But CoQ$_{10}$ can also fight cancer directly, through a number of different actions.

- It scavenges cancer causing free radicals.

- It stimulates the immune system (the immune connection).

- It inhibits tumor assocated cytokines.

- And in two studies of breast cancer patients, CoQ$_{10}$ supplementation led to a dramatic regression of cancer.[8]

  Recommended dosage: 200–800 mg per day divided into two or three doses.

Artemisinin

Artemisinin is an alkaloid of the sweet wormwood plant (*Artemisia annua*) that has long been used to treat malaria and parasites. But it turns out to also have direct anti-cancer activity. Cancer cells need a high concentration of iron in order to divide and grow. Artemisinin reacts with that iron to form free radicals that kill the cancer cells.

Artemisinin is most effective for treating colon cancer and leukemia, but it can also effectively treat quite a few other cancers (brain, breast, ovarian, prostate, and renal cancers, as well as melanoma).

- In a study conducted by Narenda Singh at the University of Washington, artemisinin killed 75 percent of breast-cancer cells in vitro after just eight hours of exposure. After twenty-four hours of exposure, almost 100 percent of the cells had been killed.[9]

- Artemisinin can be combined with other natural remedies or off-use drugs in different treatment protocols. It works well in combination with germanium-132 and L-carnitine, and is used with poly-MVA to treat brain cancer.

- High doses of oxygen significantly enhance artemisinin's ability to kill cancer cells. In a 2010 study, researchers at the University of Washington tested artemisinin alone and together with hyperbaric oxygen therapy (HBOT—*see* Chapter 6) on a culture of human leukemia cells. Using artemisinin or HBOT alone reduced cancer cell growth by 15 percent. Using them together reduced it by 38 percent.[10]

Taking artemisinin. Investigators have found that the body sometimes metabolizes artemisinin so rapidly that sufficient blood levels of the substance can't be achieved. Or sometimes the blood level gets too high. In either case, stop taking artemisinin for one to eight days.

- If the level is too low, take 15–25 mg per kg of body weight per day of DCA (dichloroacetic acid—*see* Chapter 7) during this break in order to build up your level of 5-aminolevulinic acid (5-ALA), a chemical that artemisinin uses to bind to iron.

- If the level is too high, wait until it drops.

The dose of artemisinin is 1,000 mg per day. Take the capsules orally with plain yogurt or feta cheese (for better absorption and to prevent upset stomach), along with 3 grams each of the omega-3 fatty acids EPA and DHA.

Do not take artemisinin *either* two months before *or* two months after radiation therapy.

Vitamin C

To avoid repetition, I'll just refer you back to Chapter 3, which explained that vitamin C is a fantastic, powerful, and inexpensive natural cytotoxic agent. Take vitamin C orally even if you're getting high-dose intravenous vitamin C.

The recommended dosage for cancer patients starts at 5,000 mg per day and can go up to 20,000 mg per day. You take it to bowel tolerance, which means that at a certain dosage level you will develop diarrhea. Take the highest dose that *doesn't* give you diarrhea. If you're taking the powder form, buffered C is preferable, to protect your stomach.

PectaSol

This product, invented by Dr. Isaac Eliaz, is a modified version of pectins found in citrus fruit. A study at Columbia University Medical Center tested the ability of modified citrus pectins (MCP) to induce apoptosis and inhibit cell growth in prostate cancer cell lines. After four days of treatment with a 1 percent solution of PectaSol, the percentage of cancer cells destroyed ranged from 23 percent to 52.2 percent. In the same study, PectaSol also reduced lung metastasis in rats with prostate cancer.[11]

In human patients, MCP increases the PSA doubling time (the time it takes for prostate-specific antigen levels in the blood to increase by 100 percent, an indicator of prostate cancer progression). Increasing this doubling time slows the progression of the cancer.

Recommended dosage: There are two versions, PectaSol and PectaSol-C. I recommend PectaSol-C, which is slightly more potent. Dissolve a 5 gram scoop of powder in water, juice, or tea. Don't stir; let the mixture sit three to five minutes, then stir until the powder dissolves.

Garlic

No doubt you already know that garlic (the stinking rose, as it's been called) has many health benefits. Garlic's chemistry is quite complex, but research has shown that the organosulfur compounds it contains are mainly responsible for its therapeutic properties. The most important of these compounds is allicin.

Allicin is not present in undamaged, uncrushed garlic. Fresh cloves contain the organosulfur alliin and a high level of the enzyme alliinase, stored in separate compartments of the clove. When garlic is crushed, alliinase acts on alliin and produces allicin within seconds. Allicin, in turn, breaks down rapidly to form a number of organosulfur compounds. These substances are far more stable and are responsible for allicin's health benefits.

Garlic is used to treat many diseases. For cancer, it has two uses.

- *Prevention.* Garlic is antitumorigenic (it prevents tumors from developing) and antimutagenic (it prevents mutations).

- *Treatment.* Garlic fights tumors by preventing cell mutations.

The recommended dosage is 1,000–1,500 mg of garlic powder, taken in capsules, per day.

Caution: Garlic has a blood-thinning effect, so if you are taking warfarin, coumadin, or any other anticoagulant, observe carefully whether you develop any signs of bleeding, such as blood in your stool or urine, bruises, or nosebleeds. If any such signs appear, decrease the amount of garlic you take.

Melatonin

Melatonin is a hormone produced naturally by the pineal gland in the brain. Synthetic melatonin can be taken as a supplement. Melatonin has a number of anti-cancer properties.

- It has powerful antioxidant activity.

- It may increase survival time for cancer patients.

- It inhibits angiogenesis.

- Many cancer cells have melatonin receptors. When you take melatonin, these receptors take it in, and it makes the cells inactive.

Recommended dosage: 20 mg per day, taken in one or two doses.

Zyflamend

This well-researched formula contains ten herbal extracts. Early lab studies have shown that Zyflamend has a strong cytotoxic effect and can induce apoptosis. Researchers at the MD Andersen Cancer Center found that Zyflamend has antiangiogenetic, antioxidant, antiproliferation, and apoptotic abilities.

Zyflamend also has considerable anti-inflammatory properties (inflammation connection). In two studies, it decreased the activity of proinflammatory COX and LOX enzymes that caused carcinogenesis in oral and in prostate cancer.[12]

Zyflamend contains holy basil (known as *tulsi* in ayurvedic medicine), rich in ursolic acid, which may enhance detoxification and promote a healthy response to inflammation. In addition, it contains Baikal skullcap (*Scutellaria baicalensis*), barberry, Chinese goldthread, ginger, green tea, hu zheng (*Polygonum cuspidatum,* an herb rich in resveratrol), oregano, rosemary, and turmeric.

Recommended dosage: two softgels twice a day.

THE INFLAMMATION CONNECTION— NATURAL ANTI-INFLAMMATORY SUBSTANCES

Artemisinin, melatonin, quercetin, and resveratrol, described in the previous section as cytotoxic substances addressing the genetic connection, also have considerable anti-inflammatory properties. And Zyflamend, described above, contains ten anti-inflammatory herbs and is also excellent for addressing the inflammation connection.

Inflamma Guard

In my practice I use my own formula, Inflamma Guard, which can block multiple inflammatory pathways. It contains proteolytic enzymes (including serrapeptase) that break down inflammatory proteins, as well as boswellia, ginger, hu zheng, quercetin, resveratol, rosemary, rutin, and turmeric.

- Ginger, quercetin, resveratrol, and turmeric inhibit COX-2.

Unlike aspirin or other NSAIDs, Inflamma Guard inhibits COX-1 only minimally, which is very important for avoiding blood thinning and gastrointestinal irritation, as well as for proper functioning of many body tissues, including the kidneys and the intestinal cells.

- Inflamma Guard has a mild antithrombotic (blood-thinning) effect. There are three reasons for this.

  1. There is minimal COX-1 inhibition by ginger and resveratrol.

  2. There is a mild anticoagulating activity of quercetin and turmeric.

  3. There is also fibrinolytic activity (reducing clumping of blood platelets, which prevents blood clots) of proteolytic enzymes, including serrapeptase. Fibrinolytic activity may reduce the risk of cancer proliferation and metastasis.

- Inflamma Guard may be superior to selective COX-2 inhibitors, such as Celebrex and Vioxx, for three reasons.

  1. Selective COX-2 inhibitors don't inhibit COX-1. Inhibiting COX-1 is especially important for anyone who consumes few omega-3 fatty acids and has low levels of these beneficial fats (which inhibit COX-1).

  2. Boswellia, turmeric, ginger, quercetin, and resveratrol inhibit the LOX enzyme, while the COX-2 inhibitors do not.

  3. Inflamma Guard blocks many different inflammatory pathways at the same time, whereas many anti-inflammatory drugs block only one pathway. For example, VIOXX and Celebrex block only COX-2. When COX-2 is blocked, the inflammation simply takes the LOX-1 pathway, which leads to bronchospams and asthma.

Ginger and turmeric can block phospholipase A2 (PLA2), and quercetin can block the proinflammatory substances tumor-necrosis factor–alpha (TNF-alpha). This means that Inflamma Guard has anti-inflammatory actions similar to those of corticosteroid drugs, but without any side effects.

- When taken with food, the proteolytic enzymes in Inflamma Guard assist protein digestion, reducing the chance of allergic reactions to food. This prevents any inflammatory response to undigested proteins, such as casein (milk protein), egg, gluten, or soy, and may reduce the amount of inflammation in the body as a whole.

For people with cancer, I recommend two capsules twice a day with food.

Methylsulfonylmethane (MSM)

Another great natural anti-inflammatory agent is MSM, an incredible form of sulfur. MSM actually has a wide range of effects, for it also helps the body maintain the correct pH and is critical to the formation of glutathione, which is essential for the immune system to function at peak efficiency.

Recommended dosage: A person with cancer requires 20g per day of MSM, which amounts to 40 capsules a day. Alternatively, you can take one heaping teaspoon of powder (5 g) four times a day. It's advisable to take MSM with 3,000–5,000 mg of vitamin C and 3,000–5,000 mcg of vitamin B_{12} daily.

Cayenne Pepper

This hot red pepper is not just a culinary seasoning but a great medicinal herb. A number of organizations, including the American Association of Cancer Research, have recommended it as an effective natural anti-cancer substance. A study conducted at Cedars-Sinai Medical Center found that capsaicin, cayenne's main active ingredient, caused human prostate cancer cells to undergo apoptosis and also reduced their growth rate.[13]

Several anecdotal reports suggest that cayenne has powerful anti-inflammatory and immune stimulating abilities. It also increases blood circulation, bringing more oxygen to the cancer cells. As you know, cancer cells thrive in areas where circulation is inadequate. In this way, cayenne also addresses the oxygen connection. And because it's also an alkalyzing agent, cayenne addresses the pH connection.

Suggested dosage: up to one teaspoon of cayenne powder in a glass of water, three times per day, with food.

THE OXYGEN CONNECTION

Germanium-132

In 1967, the late Dr. Kazuohiko Asai was able to synthesize germanium-132, a form of organically bound germanium, which brings oxygen to healthy tissues. Each atom of germanium-132 is bonded to three oxygen atoms, making it an efficient oxygen carrier. According to Stephen A. Levine, Ph.D., germanium can partially substitute for oxygen therapy. It improves oxygen utilization at the cellular level—which, as you know, is deadly for cancer cells. Dr. Asai found germanium-132 to be effective for treating bladder, breast, larynx, and lung cancer, plus leukemia. Germanium is also an excellent immune enhancer (*see* Breaking the Immune Connection, below).

Recommended dosage: eight to ten 250 mg capsules per day.

Methylsulfonylmethane (MSM)

This form of sulfur is the third most common chemical in the body. It makes cancer cells permeable in the same way that insulin does, so it helps treat cancer by opening the gates for another cytotoxic agent to enter these cells. In addition to being an anti-inflammatory agent, MSM also oxygenates the blood, enabling it to deliver more oxygen to the cells, just as UVA-B does. MSM increases lung capacity, meaning you can take in more oxygen.

Recommended dosage: A person with cancer requires 20g per day of MSM, which amounts to 40 capsules a day. Alternatively you can take one heaping teaspoon of powder (5 g) four times a day. It's advisable to take MSM with 3,000–5,000 mg per day of vitamin C and 3,000–5,000 mcg of vitamin B_{12} daily.

Pawpaw

This tree native to North America (*Asimina triloba*) is a cousin of graviola. According to Dr. Jerry McLaughlin, who researched and tested it in human studies, it's a far more potent anti-cancer remedy than graviola. Pawpaw works by modifying the cell's energy producing process. Whereas normally the final product is energy and water, when pawpaw is present the final product is energy and hydrogen peroxide. And you know from Chapter 6 how hydrogen peroxide fights cancer.

Recommended dosage: 50 mg per day divided into two doses of two 12.5-mg capsules.

Cautions:

- Do not take pawpaw with CoQ_{10}, any kind of thyroid medication, or superoxide dismutase.

- Do not take any antioxidants when taking pawpaw.

Rhodiola Rosea and Rhododendron Caucasicum

Both these plants, which grow in cold climates, are extremely effective adaptogens (herbs that enable the body to resist stress). Both address multiple cancer connections—genetic, oxygen, obesity, and stress.

- Both contain bioflavonoids with strong antioxidant effects (oxygen connection).

- Both raise dopamine levels and stimulate serotonin production. Increasing these two neurotransmitters eases the depression and anxiety that are so common in people with cancer (stress connection). Raising the levels of these neurotransmitters is a component of weight-loss programs (obesity connection), because when people are anxious and depressed, they eat.

- Both inhibit tumor growth and metastasis (genetic connection).

Suggested dosage: Two 250 mg capsules, twice a day.

THE SUGAR CONNECTION: NORMALIZING SUGAR LEVELS NATURALLY

Because there are so many natural substances that can maintain normal sugar levels, the only realistic approach to addressing abnormal sugar levels with nutritional supplementation is to use a synergistic combination of substances. I use two such formulas.

Gluco Guard

Gluco Guard contains nine well-researched nutrients that help maintain healthy glucose levels. This formula reduces sugar cravings and helps cells take in and burn glucose. Two capsules contain the following:

- Chromium polynicotinate (300 mg), which functions as the Glucose Tolerance Factor (GTF; a complex required for normal glucose tolerance). This complex attaches insulin to cell-membrane receptor sites.

- Cinnamon extract (500 mg). A 2003 study found that cinnamon reduces blood sugar levels and improves insulin sensitivity.[14]

- *Gymnema sylvestre* leaf extract (200 mg), yielding 50 mg of gymnemic acid. This well-known sugar-lowering herb contains phytonutrients (beneficial plant substances) that help normalize blood sugar levels and insulin production.

- Alpha-lipoic acid (150 mg). A potent antioxidant that helps inhibit glycation. Glycation is a process by which a protein or lipid molecule binds with a sugar molecule, such as glucose, forming a tangled mass of tissue. The glycated tissue becomes tough and inflexible and starts producing glycotoxins, substances that damage healthy cells, produce free radicals, and increase inflammation. Glycation is clearly part of the sugar connection. In fact, one way to treat it is to keep sugar intake low.

- L-taurine (150 mg). An amino acid that helps remove triglycerides from the bloodstream and reduce sugar cravings. It also assists the release of insulin.

- Green tea (72 mg). I've described many benefits of EGCG in the section on tea. Still another is that it augments the beneficial metabolic, vascular, and anti-inflammatory actions of insulin.

The next three ingredients are all necessary for effective processing and utilization of insulin:

- Vitamin B_6 (4.5 mg)

- Vitamin B_{12} (methylcobalamin, 75 mcg)

- Biotin (1,000 mcg)

Recommended dosage: one capsule of Gluco Guard twice a day.

Blood Sugar Guard

Four capsules of this formula contain:

- *Gymnema sylvestre* (400 mg)

- Cinnamon (400 mg)

- *Salacia oblonga* extract (500 mg). This herb has long been used in ayurvedic medicine to manage diabetes and obesity. It is reported to improve type 2 diabetes and hyperglycemia associated with obesity.

- Fenugreek (500 mg). Laboratory and human studies indicate that this herb, used in ayurvedic and Chinese medicine, can help lower blood sugar, especially when combined with other substances.

- American ginseng (*Panax quinquefolium,* 400 mg) has been found to lower blood sugar in people with type 2 diabetes, both on an empty stomach and after eating.

- Banaba (*Lagerstroemia speciosa,* 400 mg). Like insulin, banaba leaf extract induces the transport of glucose from the bloodstream into cells; it lowers blood sugar in people with type 2 diabetes.

- Kudzu (*Pueraria lobata,* 400 mg) is a vine originally from Asia that grows wild in the southeastern U.S. Research indicates that it can improve insulin resistance, a precursor to type 2 diabetes.

Suggested dosage: two capsules of Blood Sugar Guard twice a day with meals.

Both Gluco Guard and Blood Sugar Guard also address the MID and obesity connections.

THE MID CONNECTION

Quite a few supplements address the MID connection. Both Gluco Guard and Blood Sugar Guard regulate insulin, sugar, and lipid metabolism, thus helping reverse metabolic immunodepression. Garlic, too, is excellent for reducing the levels of lipids in the blood, which means that it too reverses MID.

Lipid Guard

Another formula I use to address MID is Lipid Guard, which combines two nutrients that maintain cholesterol at healthy levels. One capsule contains:

- Policosanol (10 mg), a blend of natural plant wax extracts that lowers LDL (bad) cholesterol and increases HDL (good) cholesterol.

- Gugulipid (490 mg), an extract from the resin of an Indian plant, gum guggul (*Commiphora mukul*). Guggul's active ingredients safely maintain normal cholesterol and triglyceride levels without depleting the body's CoQ_{10} supply the way statin drugs do.

Suggested dosage: one capsule three times a day.

Pantethine and Pantothenic Acid

When pantothenic acid (vitamin B_5) enters the body, it is converted into pantethine. Pantethine, in turn, is converted into coenzyme A, which is needed for generating energy from fats, carbohydrates, and proteins. Coenzyme A is also required for synthesizing fats, cholesterol, the neurotransmitter acetylcholine, melatonin, and the steroid hormones.

Pantethine may also reduce the body's synthesis of cholesterol. Since both pantethine and pantothenic acid support lipid and sugar metabolism, they play an important role in reversing MID. They work better in combination.

Recommended dosages: pantothenic acid, 500 mg once a day, pantethine, 250 mg three times a day. You can find formulas that include both nutrients.

TAKING CARE OF THE OBESITY CONNECTION

Addressing obesity in the early stages of cancer is absolutely essential. You must look at losing weight as a form of prevention that keeps the cancer from progressing. Weight loss begins with Gluco Guard and Blood Sugar Guard. Next, a number of fat-burning amino acids come in handy.

Amino Acids

Amino acids are the building blocks of proteins, and they perform many other duties as well, including burning fat for weight loss.

Glutamine, Arginine, and Glycine

The amino acids *glutamine, arginine,* and *glycine* stimulate production of fat-burning hormones, including somatotropin, the growth hormone.

Glutamine is one of the most prescribed supplements. It stimulates production of fat-burning hormones (e.g. human growth hormone), stabilizes blood sugar, and decreases sugar cravings. When blood sugar is low, glutamine decreases production of insulin, in order to prevent hypoglycemia, and stimulates production of glycogen (a form of glucose that is stored in the liver and muscles). The glycogen can then be released into the blood to bring the low sugar level up to normal. Glutamine is also involved in the liver's synthesis of glutathione, an important antioxidant that many integrative physicians use in treating certain cancers. Recommended dosage: 9,000–15,000 mg divided into three doses.

Arginine. This amino acid contributes significantly to insulin production and regulation of lipid metabolism. It can enhance the ratio of lean tissue to body fat, thereby helping you control weight. Recommended dosage: 1,500–2,000 mg divided into three doses.

Glycine is particularly useful in the form of dimethylglycine (DMG), which has been found to lower blood cholesterol, triglyceride, and glucose levels (thus also addressing the MID connection). It helps maintain low weight. Recommended dosage: 500 mg three times a day.

Carnitine

This compound, found in most body tissues, helps turn fat into energy. Carnitine transports fatty acids rapidly into cells and, metaphorically speaking, throws them into the metabolic "oven" of the mitochondria, so the body burns fat instead of storing it. That's why you will see it referred to as a fat burner. A 2004 study found that taking carnitine can move fatty acids more rapidly out of fat cells (adipocytes) and increase oxidation of fatty acids left in those cells.[15] And in a number of animal studies, carnitine supplementation during a low-calorie diet resulted in a significant decrease in body fat, compared to animals who got placebos.[16]

Recommended dosage: 3,000 mg of L-carnitine, divided into three doses. (L-carnitine is the biologically active form used as a supplement.)

Even while taking carnitine supplements, you must also maintain your body's ability to synthesize carnitine. This synthesis requires the presence of vitamin B_6, vitamin B_{12}, vitamin B_3 (niacin), and folic acid. In order to function properly, carnitine also requires the complete vitamin B complex, along with zinc-containing enzymes that are needed to synthesize growth hormone, thyroid hormone, and sex hormones—all important in weight management.

Hoodia Gordonii

Hoodia is a succulent plant native to southern Africa. A small amount of research backs up anecdotal claims that hoodia is an appetite suppressant. Researchers have suggested that hoodia releases a chemical similar to glucose that tricks the brain into believing that the stomach is full. My own experience with hoodia is inconclusive. It works for some people but not for others.

Recommended dosage: 3,000–4,500 mg per day divided into two or three doses.

THE PH CONNECTION—IS IT MANAGEABLE?

Spectographic and isotope studies of cell membranes have shown that tumor cells like to absorb the alkaline minerals cesium, rubidium, and potassium. The presence of the antioxidants vitamin C and zinc enhances the cancer cell's ability to take in these minerals. Thus one way to manage the pH connection is to administer these substances, with the goal of making the cancer cells more alkaline.

Cesium (in the form of cesium chloride) or rubidium (in the form of rubidium chloride) can change a cancer cell in two ways.

1. They limit the cell's uptake of glucose, essentially starving it (sugar connection).

2. They raise the pH inside the cell to approximately 8.0—a deadly level. In fact, cancer cells die within forty-eight to seventy-two hours in such an alkaline environment.

There is a second explanation for the effects of cesium chloride and rubidium chloride (cesium is used much more often than rubidium). According to this theory, glucose is transported across the cancer cell membrane into the cell by a biochemical mechanism called the sodium-potassium pump, which moves sodium out of the cell and potassium into it. In order to bring in the amount of glucose that the cancer cell needs, the pump must function twenty times faster than normal. Conveniently enough, cesium acts like potassium, and when it is present, great quantities of it are pumped right into the cell. Once inside the cell, the cesium blocks the pump's outbound channel, which means the cesium can't get out and builds up inside the cell. The theory suggests that this built-up cesium kills the cells by an unknown mechanism.

In 1984, Keith Brewer, Ph.D. successfully treated thirty people who had cancer with cesium chloride. H.P. Sartori conducted a study from 1981–1984 at Life Science Universal Medical Center in Rockland, MD, and Washington, D.C. He gave fifty patients 6–9g of cesium chloride a day (an extremely high dose), divided into three equal doses. They ate a special diet consisting mainly of whole grains, vegetables, linseed, walnuts, soy, and wheat germ. They also took vitamin A (100,000 IU), vitamin C (4,000–30,000 mg), zinc (40–100 mg), selenium (600–1,200 mcg), laetrile (1,500 mg), and some vitamin K and magnesium salts. As of July 1984, twenty-five of these people (who had been expected to die within two weeks to three months after treatment began in 1981), had survived for three years and three months. What was more, their pain disappeared one to three days after cesium therapy began.

Achieving a pH level of 8.0 is quite difficult, however. It's easier said than done. And some people's bodies are calcium-deficient, in which case it's impossible to increase the pH in their cells by more than 0.1 or 0.2, certainly not to 8.0. This is because when the body is calcium deficient, it tries to stay acidic in order to extract calcium from food. Of course you don't want the body to be acidic, since that makes the cancer cells very happy, so such people can't use this treatment.

All cesium and rubidium chloride treatments also require taking up to 500 mg per day of potassium.

My take on cesium/rubidium therapy:

- The fact that it works for some patients doesn't mean it will work for everyone;

- Cesium/rubidium therapy may not be the best treatment for certain types or stages of cancer;

- It's not always known if someone's body will be able to reach a pH of 8.0. In fact, I believe this is possible only theoretically. In practice, it's impossible.

Personally, I prefer Mark Rosenberg's protocol (*see* Chapter 7) for managing the pH connection (and interestingly, this protocol works in the opposite way, by making the cells extremely acidic instead of extremely alkaline). While cesium and rubidium can be administered more easily than Rosenberg's program, I consider his protocol more useful and practical, especially since it's so difficult to raise the pH of a cell to 8.0.

BREAKING THE IMMUNE CONNECTION

Any alternative cancer-care book will tell you that the paramount issue in treatment is stimulating the immune system of the person with cancer. That's an important, true statement. But I'd add that boosting the immune system is actually only one among *ten* paramount issues. That is, addressing the immune connection is no more important than addressing every other cancer connection.

Quite a few nutritional supplements can address the immune system, and in my opinion, taking each of them separately isn't practical. I prefer a synergistic formula. As you'll see from the list that follows, mother nature has provided more than enough weapons to address the immune connection. The main thing is to start right away, and do it right.

Immuno Guard

My proprietary formula Immuno Guard contains thirteen natural substances that have been found to stimulate natural killer cells, cytokine synthesis, and T- and B-cell responses.

- *Echinacea augustifolia* (300 mg). This common North American plant has been found to boost resistance to illness, apparently through its effects on the immune system.

- Goldenseal (*Hydrastis canadensis,* 100 mg). Research suggests that goldenseal, like echinacea, enhances immune function.

- Green tea (300 mg). In addition to all its other cancer-fighting abilities, research indicates that green tea improves the functioning of natural killer (NK) cells.

- Astragalus (*Astragalus membranaceus,* 200 mg) is an adaptogen long used in Chinese medicine. It has been shown to stimulate the immune system in a number of ways.

- Elderberry (*Sambucus nigra,* 200 mg) is commonly used worldwide to stimulate the immune system in cases of colds and flu.

- *Andrographis paniculata* (200 mg) is commonly used in Asia as an immune support.

- Larch tree (100 mg) contains a compound called arabinogalactan that can stimulate the action of natural killer cells and enhance other immune functions.

- Fungi (50 mg each): *Cordyceps sinensis,* a fungus that grows on caterpillars; and reishi (*Ganoderma lucidum*), shiitake (*Lentinus edodes*), and maitake (*Grifola frondosa*) mushrooms all stimulate immune function.

- Monolaurin (lauric acid, 100 mg), a fatty acid found in coconut oil, stimulates production of T cells.

- Beta 1,3 glucan (9 mg). Beta-glucans, substances found in the cell walls of many mushrooms, have immune-boosting properties. Beta 1, 3 glucan is the most active form.

Recommended dosage: one capsule, three times a day.

MGN-3

This patented supplement consists of rice bran and mushroom extracts. It is based on six years of research, which found that it increased the production of natural killer cells.

Recommended dosage: four capsules three times per day for three weeks. Then take a maintenance level of four capsules a day. For best results, take MGN-3 two hours before or two hours after taking other supplements.

PSK

Another mushroom extract containing complex polysaccharides (a type of carbohydrate). This very potent immune stimulator has been used for years in Japan and extensively researched. Although I myself use Immuno Guard, other experts report that PSK can definitely be used to break the immune connection.

Recommended dosage: 200 mg per day divided into two doses.

Germanium-132

This synthetic form of the mineral germanium is one of the best nutritional cancer treatments. It is an immune enhancer and inhibits tumor growth. It also causes a decrease in metastasis, prolongs survival time, and helps people gain weight lost due to chemo treatments.

Recommended dosage: eight to ten 250 mg capsules per day.

Phycotene

This product contains seventeen carotenoids (the substances that give carrots and sweet potatos their color) extracted from the algae spirulina and dunaliella. They include beta-carotene, which is a powerful antioxidant and may play a role in scavenging free radicals, as well as helping protect normal cells.

Recommended dosage: one capsule twice a day.

Avemar

Avemar is a fermented wheat germ product that supports healthy immune function and helps cells differentiate and repair properly. Many laboratory, animal, and clinical studies have shown that Avemar regulates glucose metabolism in the cell and promotes the ability of white blood cells to target and kill cancer cells. Many integrative physicians use Avemar and report success.

Recommended dosage: Avemar comes in individual packets. Use one packet each day. Dissolve the powder in water and drink.

RELEASING THE STRESS CONNECTION

When you're confronting cancer, there's no such thing as a minor issue. Every issue is a major issue, especially when it involves the cancer connections. And the stress connection is no exception. You can break all the cancer connections, but if you don't relieve stress, watch out. You're destined to fail.

I address the stress connection using amino acids and two of my own formulas: Stress Guard and Adrenal Guard. But there's more to addressing stress than taking supplements, and Chapter 10 describes essential lifestyle measures that enable you to de-stress.

Stress Guard

Stress Guard is a synergistic formula that includes gamma-aminobutyric acid (GABA), the most important calming neurotransmitter. GABA prevents nerve signals that transmit anxiety and stress from reaching the brain. Each capsule of this formula contains the following nutrients.

- GABA (300 mg)
- Glycine (useful for calming as well as weight loss, 200 mg)
- Niacin (100 mg)
- Pantothenic acid (100 mg)
- Vitamin B$_6$ (10 mg)

  Recommended dosage: one capsule a day.

Adrenal Guard

The supplements in this formula relieve adrenal-gland exhaustion resulting from chronic stress. Two capsules contain the following.

- Vitamin C (100 mg)

- Vitamin B_1 (2 mg)

- Vitamin B_2 (5 mg)

- Vitamin B_6 (5 mg)

- Pantothenic acid (250 mg)

- Whole adrenal glandular (extract of adrenal gland tissue, 200 mg)

- PABA (para-aminobenzoic acid, part of vitamin B complex, 100 mg)

- N-acetyl tyrosine (an amino acid, 50 mg)

- Adrenal cortex glandular (50 mg)

  Recommended dosage: two capsules a day with meals.

Tryptophan

This amino acid converts to the neurotransmitter serotonin, which the pineal gland in the brain converts at night into melatonin, the hormone that induces sleep. Some people also find tryptophan useful to relieve anxiety and depression.

Tryptophan may also address the obesity connection. A 1997 study found that the higher the dose of tryptophan taken an hour before a meal by obese people, the less carbohydrate they ate.[17]

Recommended dosage: 500 mg, three times a day. Take forty minutes before or after eating.

Theanine

Found mostly in the tea plant, theanine is what gives green tea a calming effect even though the tea also contains a stimulant. Research indicates that theanine stimulates production of alpha (relaxing) brain waves, and that it modulates the release of neurotransmitters, also producing a relaxation effect.

Recommended dosage: 200 mg per day, taken in one or two doses.

FINAL THOUGHTS

I know from experience that people tend to become anxious when faced with a long list of supplements like the one you've just read. So I want to reassure you that *you don't need to take all of them*. Here's how to proceed.

- *First,* choose a few of the natural cytotoxic agents (ideally, with the guidance of an experienced integrative physician).

- *Second* (again with the physician's help, if possible) determine all the cancer connections that might be present in your body. Begin addressing those connections by taking some of the supplements recommended for each one. Again, you don't need all the supplements listed—just taking my formulas will suffice. To address those connections for which there is no formula, discuss the relevant supplements with your integrative physician.

- *Third,* every two months, evaluate your supplement program using blood tests and other diagnostic tools. Make any adjustments accordingly.

Cancer doesn't sleep, so you need to stay vigilant yourself. On their first visit, many new patients assure me they don't need more supplements. They'll say, "Doc, I already take multivitamins and vitamin E. That should be enough." And I tell them, "Definitely not."

I've just warned you against oversupplementation. Now I must also warn you against *under*supplementation. Take as your basic principle that *supplementation should be adequate, balanced, and practical.*

What does this mean? Taking one or two separate vitamins won't even touch your cancer, much less prevent it from progressing. On the other hand, taking a huge, indiscriminate number of supplements will just make you sick. My patients who go down this road often get upset and give up. That's no good either.

That's why I believe the best course is to rely on an integrative physician to tell you which supplements are musts and which you can do without. But I'm aware that you may not be able to consult such a physician. If that's true for you, here's what to do.

Try to determine which cancer connections are present in your body by answering the following questions.

- Are you obese?

- Is your insulin level high?

- Do you crave sweets?

- Are your cholesterol and triglyceride levels high?

- How's your pH level? (pH testing paper is a reliable indicator to check the pH of your saliva and urine.)

- What condition is your immune system in? Do you get frequent colds or fungal infections?

- How's your stress level?

Use your answers as guides that indicate what cancer connections you need to address. Then, based on your conclusions, use the information I've provided throughout this book to put together an initial supplement program. (If you'd like to purchase some of my formulas, call 718-368-9555.)

You (and your doctor) have a lot of work cut out for you. What are you waiting for?

PART THREE

Essential Adjuncts: Detox, Diet, and Stress-Relieving Programs

By now you've gotten the idea that cancer doesn't give up easily, and a simple approach whose mission is nothing more than *Kill it* won't work. The fact is that a cancerous tumor doesn't live in outer space. It lives in an inner space—your space—that is, your body. Every aspect of its growth and other behavior affects this body in many different ways.

What's more, a body that develops cancer may already be sick with different diseases related to a poorly functioning immune system. It could be full of inflammation, or just plain toxic. In such a body, the colon, liver, and kidneys can't fully perform their responsibilities of cleansing and detoxification. Physicians can kill cancer cells as much as they like, but if the body is unable to remove the dead cells and other toxins produced by the cancer cells, it may grow even sicker. And if you don't follow an appropriate anti-cancer diet you will only introduce more toxins and exacerbate a number of the cancer connections. Instead of getting better and feeling better, you'll continue to be impaired.

From the moment you awake in the morning to the time you fall asleep at night, your body is subjected to many different forms of stress. And don't think stress vanishes while you're sleeping. Stress easily disrupts your sleep pattern, causing sleepless nights that stress your body even further.

What this means is that every single person with cancer must do everything possible to prepare the body for the great battle against the disease, by cleansing and detoxifying it and by relieving stress. These measures must be an ongoing, daily component of your anti-cancer program, part of your lifestyle. Chapters 9 and 10 will tell you how to cleanse, detoxify, and relieve stress. Please read them carefully.

CHAPTER 9

— — — ▬ — — —

Cancer Connection 9—
Toxins and How to Get Rid of Them

INITIAL THOUGHTS

The ninth cancer connection is the toxic environment that surrounds us all. This factor is so important that I'm devoting an entire chapter to it.

Most people are aware that tobacco smoke and exposure to asbestos have been strongly linked to lung cancer. These substances are widely accepted as environmental carcinogens. But they're only the tip of the environmental iceberg. A reader of this book no doubt knows there are many more. Over the years, integrative physicians around the world have learned the hard way that environmental toxins are a huge factor in cancer development.

I'm aware that the very nature of cancer biology makes it difficult to prove that the toxicity connection really exists. Cancer has a long latency period, and it's not easy to design a study that can determine someone's toxicity exposure during such a lengthy period. Nevertheless, I believe very strongly in the toxicity connection, because there is a strong correlation between a toxic environment and a high prevalence of cancer. Integrative oncologists all agree that *they have not yet seen a single patient whose cancer didn't reveal a connection to some toxic exposure.*

THE TOXICITY CONNECTION

It's a dirty world out there, full of toxins that contaminate the air you breathe, the water you drink, the food you eat, the clothes you wear, even many of the personal products you use—toothpaste, for instance. No matter how you try to rid yourself of these chemicals, heavy metals, and other toxins, they soon reappear. You may want to escape them, but you really can't.

When these toxins get inside the body, they trigger three different mechanisms that correspond to three cancer connections.

• *Inflammatory connection.* Toxins trigger inflammatory cytokine pathways.

• *Genetic connection.* Toxins trigger gene mutation.

• *Immune connection.* The gastrointestinal tract is full of immune cells, including structures called Peyer's patches whose function is to stimulate an immune response when pathogens are present. If the intestine is full of toxins, this function is impaired, and the immune defenses are weakened. (I believe, in fact, that immune stability begins in the intestine and bowel. That's why colon cleansing is so important—*see* below.)

Many different environmental exposures have been linked to specific types of cancer—for example, asbestos to lung cancer; benzidine, a chemical found in more than 250 dyes used in the textile industry in the past, to bladder cancer; and benzene to leukemias. Government agencies have noted the many connections between chemical exposures and cancer. In 2010, the President's Cancer Panel released a report that pulled no punches. Americans face "grievous harm" from environmental toxins that have gone unregulated, wrote the panel's experts. Outdated standards, insufficient funding for research, and weak laws have resulted in an "unacceptable burden of cancer resulting from environmental and occupational exposures that could have been prevented through appropriate national action." The previously accepted figure, that chemicals and other toxins cause only around 5 percent of cancers, is "grossly underestimated," they added.[1] And according to the National Cancer Institute (NCI) and National Institute of Environmental Health Sciences, "Exposure to a wide variety of natural and man-made substances in the environment accounts for at least two-thirds of all the cases of cancer in the United States."[2]

Two-thirds. That's a lot more than 5 percent. But it's no surprise when you consider that, according to the President's panel, only 200 of the 80,000 chemicals currently being used in the U.S. have been tested for safety, and many that are known or suspected to be carcinogenic are unregulated. As LaSalle D. Leffall Jr., M.D., the panel chair, put it, "The increasing number of known or suspected environmental carcinogens compels us to action, even though we may currently lack irrefutable proof of harm."

Of course there were naysayers. Michael J. Thun, M.D., of the American Cancer Society (ACS) asserted that the report was "unbalanced by its implication that pollution is the major cause of cancer," although he acknowledged that environmental toxins are "of particular concern." Here I must point out that ACS has a political position on cancer. This organization is unfriendly to alternative medicine and refuses to accept the need for detoxification. Therefore it must deny that toxins are a major cause of cancer.

Never mind the ACS. This chapter will provide you with an entire program of actions you can take to protect yourself.

IT'S A TOXIC, TOXIC, TOXIC WORLD

Contemporary *Homo sapiens* have become a final destination for all types of toxins, coming from anywhere and everywhere. Products that deliver these toxins to your body lurk in your kitchen and bathroom, your workplace or school. You bring them home from your dry cleaner. They emanate from your microwave, your carpets and shining floors, even the ceiling. You encounter them in your car, on trains and airplanes, and in the form of electromagnetic fields generated by your computer and cell phone. Escaping them is truly *mission impossible.* Even going out into the fresh air to play a round of golf isn't safe, given the heavy insecticide spraying that makes the golf course velvety green. In fact, golf course superintendents and frequent golfers develop 1.75 times more colon cancer, twice as much non-Hodgkin's lymphoma and brain cancer, and three times more prostate cancer than the national average.[3]

It's also scary to think about what's in the air everyone breathes. City air is absolutely toxic. It causes a tenfold increase in cancer.

- The death rate from cancer is highest in the cities with the most air pollution.

- Studies of U.S. air samples revealed that 90 percent of them contained the insecticides diazanon and DDT (which had been banned thirty years before!), 70 percent contained the insecticide chlorpyrifos (Dursban), and 60 percent contained the herbicide 2,4-D.[4]

Following is a rundown of major environmental toxins implicated in cancer.

Pesticides

About 900 active ingredients are used in pesticides in the U.S., of which 20 were found to be carcinogenic in animals. Based on these animal studies, the Environmental Protection Agency (EPA) considers 60 percent of herbicides, 30 percent of insecticides, and 90 percent of fungicides in common use to be carcinogens or potential carcinogens.[5]

Pilots who spray insecticides on crop fields are at high risk of leukemia and pancreatic cancer.[6] Exposure to 2,4-D, an ingredient of weed and feed products commonly used on lawns, is linked to leukemia when the exposure occurred during pregnancy or childhood. This chemical has also been associated with lymphomas and in fact is banned in Quebec, Sweden, Denmark, and Norway.[7] According to data from the National Cancer Institute, pesticides are linked to medulloblastomas in children born in the fall (whose mothers were pregnant during the spring and summer when crops were sprayed).

A number of pesticides have been banned, or their use restricted, in this country, including amitrole, DDT, dimethylhydrazine, ethylene oxide, lindane, and mirex. Nevertheless, the scope of pesticide residual problems is staggering: 1.2 billion pounds were dumped on American forests, fields, and lawns.[8]

Industrial Toxins

Large amounts of highly toxic chemicals and heavy metals are released every day by industry and find their way into the human body. Heavy metals such as aluminum, arsenic, cadmium, lead, mercury, and nickel can accumulate in the brain, bones, fatty tissues, glands, hair, and nerve cells, where they cause damage. The fact that the locations of toxic-waste dumpsites closely correlate with areas that have the highest rates of breast cancer mortality is good evidence of the toxicity connection.[9] So is another fact: by 1980 the EPA had detected over 400 toxic chemicals in different human tissues—48 in fat tissue, 40 in breast milk, 73 in the liver, and 250 in the blood.

Heavy Metals Heavily Linked to Cancer

Exposure to metals—especially heavy metals—can lead to different cancers. Table 9.1 lists toxic metals that many people are commonly exposed to.

TABLE 9.1. METAL CARCINOGENS			
METAL / CANCERS	PRESENT IN	HUMAN CARCINOGEN?	WORKERS EXPOSED
ARSENIC			
Skin, lung, bladder, kidney, liver	Wood preservatives, glass, pesticides	Yes	Smelting of ores containing arsenic, pesticide application, and wood preservation
BERYLLIUM			
Lung	Nuclear weapons, rocket fuel, ceramics, glass, plastic, fiber optic products	Yes	Beryllium ore miners and alloy makers, phosphor manufacturers, ceramic workers, missile technicians, nuclear reactor workers, electric and electronic equipment workers, and jewelers
CADMIUM			
Lung	Metal coatings, plastic products, batteries, fungicides	Yes	Smelting of zinc and lead ores, producing, processing and handling cadmium powders, welding or remelting of cadmium-coated steel, and working with solders that contain cadmium

METAL / CANCERS	PRESENT IN	HUMAN CARCINOGEN?	WORKERS EXPOSED
CHROMIUM			
Lung	Automotive parts, floor covering, paper, cement, asphalt roofing, anti-corrosive metal plating	Yes	Stainless steel production and welding, chromate production, chrome plating, ferrochrome alloys, chrome pigment, and tanning industries
LEAD			
Kidney, brain	Cotton dyes, metal coating, drier in paints, varnishes, and pigment inks, certain plastics, specialty glass	Probable carcinogen	Construction work that involves welding, cutting, brazing, or blasting on lead paint surfaces; most smelter workers, including lead smelters where lead is recovered from batteries; radiator repair shops
NICKEL			
Nasal cavity, lung	Steel, dental fillings, copper and brass, permanent magnets, storage batteries, glazes	*Nickel metal:* Probable carcinogen; *Nickel compounds:* Yes	Battery makers, ceramic makers, electroplaters, enamellers, glass workers, jewelers, metal workers, nickel mine workers, refiners and smelters, paint-related workers, and welders

Cancer and the Environment: What You Need To Know, What You Can Do, published by U.S. Department of Health and Human Services, National Institutes of Health, National Cancer Institute, National Institute of Environmental Health Sciences.

Mercury—A Toxin in Your Teeth

Mercury toxicity is a story in itself, because mercury is a component of dental fillings. A definite carcinogen that can impair immune function, mercury often comprises up to 50 percent of silver fillings. A great deal of evidence proves that mercury amalgams are the major source of mercury exposure for the general public. These amalgam fillings can release mercury vapors continuously, so as long as one is in your mouth, you're inhaling mercury vapor 24/7. Once the mercury is inhaled or ingested, it's converted in the body to methylmercury, the organic form of mercury, which is 100 times more toxic than elemental mercury. Methylmercury easily crosses the blood-brain barrier and causes many problems in the nervous system, including the brain. These include Alzheimer's disease, multiple sclerosis, amyotropic lateral sclerosis (ALS, or Lou Gehrig's disease), and cancer.

Toxins in Water and Milk

Polluted, fluorinated, chlorinated water equals toxic water. That's why tapwater in the U.S. is a real health hazard. Not only is it full of pesticides and agricultural runoffs that continuously contaminate it, but according to the EPA, the tapwater used by about 30 million Americans contains lead from old plumbing pipes. In fact, one of every four public water systems is in outright violation of federal standards for tapwater.[10]

Water may contain various bacteria, gasoline solvents, industrial wastes, chemical residues, and radioactive particles, among other horrors. When public health agencies take measures to disinfect or purify drinking water, they use chlorine, which can also cause cancer. According to studies conducted by experts from Harvard University and the Medical College of Wisconsin, consumption of chlorinated drinking water causes 15 percent of rectal cancers and 9 percent of bladder cancers. Drinking chlorinated water over a long period of time carries a 38 percent greater risk for contracting rectal cancer and a 2 percent greater risk for developing bladder cancer.[11]

Fluoride has been added to drinking water (and toothpaste) since the 1950s. Yet it is a poison second in toxicity only to arsenic. Fluoride causes cancer by transforming normal cells into cancerous cells. And it can do this at a concentration as low as 1 part per million. What's more, fluoride contributes to the cancer-producing potential of other chemicals. While earlier studies reported that the incidence of oral and pharyngeal cancer rose with increased exposure to fluoride and that such exposure caused 8,000 new cases each year, a 1999 report by the Centers for Disease Control concluded that there was "no credible evidence" of an association between fluoridated drinking water and an increased risk for cancer.[12] In my opinion, however, where there's smoke, there's fire. Even the possibility of an association between cancer and fluoride should make people wary.

So think twice before you drink unfiltered tapwater.

And pay attention to the milk you drink and give your children. Dairy milk is a favorite beverage of Americans, but now, alas, much of it carries cancer-producing factors. In 1993, the FDA approved the use of recombinant bovine growth hormone (rBGH), which is injected daily into dairy cattle to increase their milk production. Producing more milk is fine in itself, but—says Samuel S. Epstein, M.D., of the University of Illinois at Chicago School of Public Health—rBGH happens to contain IGF-1 (insulinlike growth factor). As the Prologue explained, IGF-1 occurs naturally in the body and causes cells to divide and grow. When an additional amount of IGF-1 enters the body in milk, the body is unable to destroy it by digestion, and it is absorbed by the colon, which has receptor sites for IGF-1. The hormone rBGH has been found to promote the growth of breast cancer cells, and no fewer than seventeen studies published since 1991 indicate that rBGH milk has cancer-producing effects. So be sure to buy non-rGBH milk.

Toxins in Food and Food Additives

Many of you are aware of the toxins in nonorganic food and already buy organic. If you aren't one of these, pay close attention. When you ingest nonorganic food, you also take in pesticides, herbicides, fungicides, and many other chemical toxins. You know now how these toxins contribute to cancer development. The same is true of many food additives. Below is a list of additives you should definitely avoid.

- *Saccharin.* Artificial sweetener found in Sweet'N Low.

- *Aspartame.* Artificial sweetener found in Equal and NutraSweet.

- *Citrus red dye no. 2.* Used to color the skins of oranges.

- *Yellow dye no. 6.* Used to color candy and sodas.

- *Monosodium glutamate.* Flavor enhancer found in processed and packaged foods as well as fast foods.

- *Brominated vegetable oil.* Used as an emulsifier in soft drinks to keep the flavor evenly distributed and give them a cloudy appearance.

- *Nitrites.* Used to preserve cured meats.

- *Butylated hydroxyanisole (BHA) and butylated hydroxytoluene (BHT).* Preservatives added to fats, oils, and foods that contain fats.

- *Tertiary butylhydroquinone.* An antioxidant added to a wide range of foods as a preservative; may be combined with other preservatives like BHA.

- *Sulfur dioxide, sodium bisulfite, sulfites.* Used to preserve shrimp, dried fruit, and frozen potatoes.

You should also be wary of the cookware, plastic containers, and cleaning products in your kitchen cabinets since they too are potential sources of toxic additives. Even organic food may be contaminated by toxins in these items. Aluminum cookware, for example, releases traces of aluminum into food. Molecules from polyvinyl chloride (PVC), polyethylene (PE), and polyvinylidene chloride (PVDC) used to make plastic containers and cling wraps migrate into food when subjected to the high temperatures in microwave ovens. And many dishwashing liquids, chlorinated powders, bleaches, all-purpose cleaners, and drain cleaners contain petrochemicals, which leave harmful chemical residues that get into food.

Irradiated Foods

Much food is now treated with ionizing radiation to kill insects, bacteria, molds and fungi, and to prevent sprouting, thereby extending shelf life. However this process could be quite damaging to health, because irradiation leads to the formation of toxic substances in the food. These include benzene, formaldelyde, and other chemical byproducts.

Food irradiation may also increase the levels of aflatoxins, cancer-causing substances produced by certain fungi that grow on foods. These fungi most commonly grow on grains and peanuts, but meat, eggs, and milk from animals that eat aflatoxin-contaminated feed can also contain aflatoxins.

Radiation

Ionizing radiation. X-ray technology and nuclear radiation from diagnostic tests using iodine-131 and other isotopes expose people to ionizing radiation. So does living or working in proximity to nuclear power plants, which can be a factor in 40 to 50 percent of cancers.

Radon is a radioactive gas formed by the natural breakdown of uranium in soil, rock, and water. It can get into any building. The EPA estimates that radon pollution may contribute to 10,000 cancers a year in the U.S.[13]

Electromagnetic Fields (EMF). Everyone today lives amid a sea of electromagnetic fields generated by the electrical wiring in homes, offices, and schools, and by cellphones, cellphone towers, computers, electrical appliances, high-voltage wires, microwave ovens, overhead lights, TVs, video terminals, and wireless computer networks. Another source of exposure is geopathic stress (produced by disturbances in the earth's natural electromagnetic fields, caused by geological formations, such as fault lines and underground water; these disturbances have harmful effects on the body).

Studies of human populations have revealed an association between EMF exposure and cancer, particularly childhood leukemia.[14] In adults, the association between EMF exposure and brain cancer is stronger.[15]

Tobacco

No need to belabor the toxic effects of tobacco, so I'll just mention two facts.

- Tobacco use causes about 400,000 cases of cancer each year in the U.S.

- About 33 percent of all cancer deaths are attributed to smoking-related lung cancer.

This list of toxins could go on, but I'm sure that by now you've got the picture.

DOUBLE D—CLEAN UP THE MESS WITH DETOX AND DIET

Living in a toxic world isn't healthy for anyone, but particularly for people who have cancer. That's why ridding your body of toxins must be your initial step in surviving the unsurvivable. Your strategy is twofold— detoxification and diet.

First D—Detox

Detoxification is not a specific anti-cancer therapy; it's an essential first step in treating not just cancer, but any chronic degenerative disease (arthritis, asthma, coronary artery disease, diabetes, and so on).

Here's my eight step detox program.

1. Balanced diet. This step is the second D (presented below), but it's also a crucial part of successful detoxing.

2. If you smoke and/or are overweight: stop smoking, lose weight.

3. Use environmentally friendly, nontoxic health and body care products and house cleaners. Use fewer plastics and avoid aluminum cookware. Also avoid furniture made of particleboard (which contains formaldehyde).

4. Colon cleansing.

5. Liver detoxification.

6. Lymphatic drainage.

7. Chelation therapy.

8. Saunas and salt baths.

Steps 2 and 3 are completely up to you, so I'll focus here on steps 4–8.

Colon Cleansing

Colon cleansing isn't a particularly palatable subject to talk about, but it's an extremely important component of detox. All the toxins being cleaned out during the detox process wind up being dumped into the colon, and if you don't clean it out, they stay in the body. The three standard methods of colon cleansing are enemas, colonics, and herbal supplements.

Enemas. This method is probably familiar to you. Choose the 2 quart water bag enema and follow the instructions on the package. But don't go overboard—be aware that enemas are habit forming and can lead to dependence, leaving you unable to move your bowels on your own. Enemas can also weaken your anal sphincter. For these reasons, it's best to rely primarily on the other two methods, especially herbal supplements.

Colonic irrigation. Like an enema, a colonic sends water up into the colon. However, it's performed by a healthcare practitioner such as a nurse or colonic therapist, using a machine. The advantage is that you lie down and relax, and the therapist does all the work by regulating the flow of water. You don't need to run to the bathroom, and the colonic cleans a larger portion of the colon than an enema does. A colonic sends about five gallons of water in and out of the colon during a forty-five minute session. Therapeutic substances, such as acidophilus, vinegar, wheatgrass, and a wide variety of herbs, can be added to the water.

Whereas someone who is severely constipated may take enemas regularly for years, you need only a short course of colonics (once or twice a week for a month or two), which you can repeat if necessary in the future.

Caution: Before starting colonics, make sure you don't have colon cancer or colon polyps, since water under pressure can cause bleeding or perforation.

Nutritional/herbal supplements. Instead of taking many enemas, use this method of cleansing often. Many bowel cleansing herbal formulas are available; look in a health food store and ask the salesperson for a recommendation.

Another excellent nutritional colon cleansing method is to take vitamin C to bowel tolerance. Take 1,000 mg every two hours until you develop diarrhea. Repeat, every other day, for ten days to two weeks.

Eliminating parasites. Treating intestinal parasites is another important part of detox. Consider asking your physician to run stool tests for parasites. If you have them, or had them in the past, you absolutely must treat them.

- Wormwood (artemisia), described in Chapter 8 as an anti-cancer herb, also has a long history of use as a *worm expeller* (hence its name). Be aware that it may initially cause your symptoms to worsen. Recommended dose: 150 mg three times a day.

- Black walnut hull is another herb that gets rid of parasites. Buy it combined with artemisia (I recommend the combo you can find at www.viable-herbal.com). Recommended dosage: one capsule twice a day during meals for two to three weeks, then once a day for another two weeks.

In all methods of colon cleansing, your goal is to clean the bowel to the point where it's practically sterile. But as you clean everything out, you must replenish the beneficial bacteria in the intestine and colon. So take probiotics every day, both during your cleanse and afterward, to restore balance in the intestinal flora.

Liver Detoxification

The liver is the major detox organ in the body, and chronic exposure to heavy metals damages both it and the kidneys, greatly impairing the body's ability to eliminate toxins. So you need to maximize your liver's ability to remove all the toxins described above from your body, as well as those caused by massive doses of chemo and radiation. Following are two practical ways to do a liver detox.

Herbal supplements containing milk thistle. This herb is a well-known liver detoxifier. Literally hundreds of studies (done mostly in Europe) have reported that milk thistle has a powerful ability to protect the liver against the effects of accidental exposures to chemical pollutants. Research has shown that silymarin, the active ingredient, significantly reduces the mortality of people with liver cirrhosis (a precancerous condition).

Recommended dosage: 200–800 mg per day. I use my own powdered formula, Green Guard, which contains many fruit and vegetable extracts plus other supplements. This combination provides antioxidant effects and support for the immune and digestive systems along with detoxification.

Coffee enemas. These are controversial, but I consider them *extremely* important. Dr. Max Gerson, creator of the Gerson diet therapy for cancer, was one of the first to use this treatment, and he advocated for it. The theory is that the coffee stimulates an enzyme system in the liver known as glutathione-S-transferase that is able to rid the bloodstream of a large number of free radicals. The reason you do an enema instead of simply drinking coffee is that the enema results in far greater absorption in the intestines. The caffeine that is absorbed goes straight to the liver, where it acts as a powerful detoxifier. According to the medical literature, the coffee enema also produces a diuretic effect, eliminating toxins by way of the urine.

Coffee enemas have been used for decades as part of Dr. Gerson's program and also in that of Dr. William Donald Kelley, a dentist who cured himself of pancreatic cancer and developed his own diet and nutritional program. Many patients who used only Gerson's diet or Kelley's raw food diet, both with coffee enemas, have been able to extend their lives.

Caution: If you want to take coffee enemas on your own, please do careful research first. Learn as much as you can about the procedure, since if you do it incorrectly and use too much coffee, you risk damaging your liver.

Use organic coffee beans, so you don't introduce new toxins with your enema, and use water that is free of fluoride or chlorine. Distilled water is best, though you can also use filtered water. Put three rounded tablespoons of drip-grind coffee in a quart of water. Boil the grounds for three minutes, then simmer fifteen to twenty minutes minutes more. Strain and cool to body temperature.

Lymphatic Drainage

The lymphatic system is a complex network of vessels and ducts that move fluids through the body. One of its main responsibilities is flushing toxins out of healthy cells. Unlike the blood circulation, the lymphatic system does not have its own pumping mechanism, and every cancer patient's lymphatic system gets extremely congested by toxins coming from a variety of sources. For this reason, using some external method to drain the lymphatic system is of paramount importance. There are two different ways to do this.

Lymphatic massage. Manual lymph drainage, a form of massage performed by a trained practitioner, was developed in the 1930s by the Danish scientist Emil Vodder. It consists of circular pumping and draining movements that move the lymph.

Light Beam Generator (LBG). This device radiates photons (light particles) that help restore the normal electromagnetic charge of cells. This change in charge enables these cells to come unstuck from other cells they are attached to. Applied to clogged lymph nodes and channels, the light penetrates deeply and enables the lymph to flow again. The equipment is a box with a long hose, at the end of which is the light beam, which the practitioner projects onto the skin. You can buy a machine, which costs around $5,000, or find a practitioner.

Chelation Therapy

Chelation is a chemical process that uses a substance to bind molecules, such as metals or minerals, and hold them tightly so they can be removed from the body. Chelation therapy is used to eliminate toxic metals and chemicals. The main chelating agent is ethylenediaminetetraacetic acid (EDTA), a synthetic amino acid that grasps the ions of heavy metals and other pollutants flooding through the bloodstream or other tissue fluids and bonds them into ringed structures so they are no longer active in the body. Or to put it more simply, the EDTA grabs hold of undesirable garbage and escorts it out of the body via the kidneys. In fact the word *chelate* is derived from the Greek *chele,* claw. Crabs and lobsters are called chelates.

Chelation also turns on all the body's repair mechanisms, leading to better, easier healing, so necessary for anyone with cancer.

- Chelation improves blood circulation.

- It delivers oxygen to cells.

- It removes poisonous compounds.

- It improves transfer of nutrients and waste materials through cell membranes.

- It increases the action of all defensive and protective mechanisms as well as offensive weapons against disease.

Other chelators are dimercaptosuccinic acid (DMSA), 2,3-dimer-capto-1-propanesulfonic acid (DMBS), and lipoic acid.

I recommend intravenous EDTA chelation therapy twice a week, for at least twenty to thirty sessions. An alternative is DMSA in oral form, 500 mg per day every other day for two months, followed by a two to four-week break and then another two-month course. During either type of treatment, your urine levels of heavy metals must be monitored, and you need a physician for this. Please do not try to be a hero and do chelation therapy on your own.

During chelation therapy you must take vitamin B_6 and zinc supplementation. Recommended dosages: B_6, 100–200 mg per day divided into two doses; zinc, 60 mg per day in two doses.

Sauna

A sauna is a very effective way to remove heavy metals and especially chemicals from the body. Chemicals and heavy metals are stored mainly in fatty tissues, and the best way to remove them is by sweating.

In my opinion the best sauna for people with cancer is an infrared sauna, which is a small unit that you can set up in your house. It uses heaters that emit radiant infrared heat, which is directly absorbed by the body. An infrared sauna doesn't produce the heavy heat that you get from a traditional sauna, which heats the body via hot air or steam. The traditional type can cause problems for people with unhealthy cardio-vascular systems—even a heart attack. The infrared sauna doesn't pose such dangers.

The sauna removes mercury and other heavy metals, including those trapped in connective tissues and the brain as well as in fat tissues. What's more, it provides pain relief by dilating blood vessels and increasing circulation to injured areas. Last, it stimulates the immune system and (like all saunas) helps you lose weight, thus addressing the immune and obesity connections.

Salt baths are a good way to remove residues from ionizing radiation. To prepare one, add sixteen ounces of Epsom salts to a warm bath and enjoy it. If you think you've been exposed to radiation, take a salt bath two to three times a week for two to three months. It will eliminate many other toxins as well. A salt bath is also a terrific muscle relaxant and fatigue reliever. If you feel exhausted at the end of the day, try one and see what it does for you.

Second D—Diet

Diet is the big second D in my detox combo. Start eating an anti-cancer diet right at the beginning of your cancer treatment program, at the same time that you begin your seven other steps of detox.

The history of alternative/integrative cancer treatment programs includes a variety of anti-cancer diets, and I see my patients become quite confused about which diet to adopt. To clear up this confusion, I'll review five well-known anti-cancer diets: the macrobiotic diet, Gerson's diet, the Budwig diet, the alkalizing diet, and the raw food diet.

Macrobiotic Diet

The word macrobiotic comes from the Greek *makro,* which means great or long, and *bios,* meaning life. Macrobiotics is more than just a diet plan, it's an entire holistic lifestyle. The theory behind using it as an anti-cancer diet is that, in addition to being free of toxins and including highly nutritional foods, it brings balance to the whole system, promoting the body's ability to heal.

The diet is mostly vegetarian and consists largely of cooked vegetables, sea vegetables, beans, and whole grains, with some fruit and small amounts of seeds, nuts, sweets, and animal foods. It also includes fermented soy products and pickles. Macrobiotic practitioners advise eating locally grown, natural foods prepared in traditional ways (baking, boiling, steaming). The diet stresses good eating habits—eating slowly and chewing food thoroughly. A potential problem with the macrobiotic diet is that without proper planning and closely following the guidelines, it can result in poor nutrition.

Gerson Diet

Max Gerson, a German physician, developed this diet, which is naturally high in vitamins, minerals, other micronutrients, and enzymes, and includes food that is low in sodium and high in potassium. In his experiments Gerson found that cancer regressed faster when people took large quantities of a potassium solution in addition to eating a high-potassium diet.

A typical daily Gerson diet consists of these components:

- Thirteen glasses of fresh raw carrot, apple, and green-leaf juices prepared hourly from fresh organic foods and vegetables;

- Three full vegetarian meals freshly prepared from organic fruits, vegetables, and whole grains—a typical meal includes a salad, cooked vegetables, a baked potato, vegetable soup, and juice;

- Fresh organic fruit, available at all hours for snacking.

In addition to adhering strictly to this diet, the following supplements are taken.

1. Potassium compound

2. Lugol's iodine solution

3. Vitamin B_{12}

4. Thyroid hormone

5. Pancreatic enzymes

In addition to the supplements, the third component of Gerson's therapy is coffee enemas. The coffee is occasionally mixed with camomile extract.

Budwig Diet

This diet was developed by Dr. Johanna Budwig, a German biochemist and expert on fats and oils, who lived to be ninety. The Budwig diet is based on a mixture of flaxseed and cottage cheese, to which other ingredients can be added to make it more palatable. You eat this combination every day along with your other food. The Budwig protocol forbids certain foods, including animal fats, other forms of dairy, any form of sugar, and all processed foods.

Alkalizing Diet

Chapter 8 described the use of cesium therapy to alkalize the body. The alkalizing diet has the same purpose. In my opinion, however, it's very difficult to raise the pH to any meaningful degree, because the body naturally tries to stay acidic in order to extract calcium from food. Used for healing, the alkalizing diet consists of 80 percent alkalizing foods and 20 percent acid-forming foods. In general, alkalizing foods include most vegetables and most (but not all) fruits. Acid-forming foods include most grains and animal proteins.

Another problem is that if you avoid some acidic foods, such as berries, you lose the benefits of their antioxidants, which I consider an important part of an anti-cancer diet.

Raw Food Diet

Raw foods play a large role in Dr. William Kelley's treatment protocol and in other anti-cancer programs. In my experience, however, cancer patients can stick to a raw-foods diet for only so long. What's more, eating some hot foods is very beneficial for digestion, and you don't get the benefit of that warmth on a raw food diet.

Dr. Yutsis' Ten Strategy Diet Program

All the diets described above have been used for decades by hundreds of people with cancer, and they've saved some lives. But following any of them successfully requires superb discipline, self control, strong motivation, and an iron will. And in real life, not everybody can do it. So I suggest to you my *realistic* diet—a healthy, balanced diet that includes the following anti-cancer strategies.

STRATEGY 1. Juice. Buy a juicer and use it daily. Drink only freshly prepared juices from organic fruits and vegetables—mainly vegetables, which are high in anti-cancer nutrients. Choose any combinations you like from among cabbage, celery, collards, kale, spinach, tomato, and wheatgrass, cayenne, dill, garlic, ginger, lemon, and tamari (these last six function as seasonings). Throughout the day, drink up to forty ounces of juice. You can add carrot and apple to your mixture to make it more palatable, but if you drink these sweet juices, I strongly advise using finger sticks to check your blood-sugar level.

STRATEGY 2. Make plant-based foods the foundation of your diet. A diet of plant-based foods can be a cancer-fighting powerhouse. Plants contain less fat than animal foods, many cancer-fighting nutrients, and, extremely important, a lot of fiber (*see* Strategy 3). Include a variety of vegetables, fruits, and whole grains, along with nuts and beans. Here's a suggested menu.

- **Breakfast.** Add fruit and a few seeds or nuts to a wholegrain cereal, such as oatmeal.

- **Lunch.** A big salad consisting of a variety of vegetables, including lots of lettuce and tomatoes, plus beans or peas. If you want a sandwich, have a veggieburger on wholegrain bread.

- **Dinner.** Replace creamy pasta sauces with fresh sautéed vegetables added to your favorite tomato sauce made with extra-virgin olive oil, and serve on brown rice. Or occasionally have a baked potato topped with broccoli and yogurt, sautéed vegetables, or salsa.

- **Snacks.** Raw vegetables with a low-fat dip, such as hummus. Or grab an apple or banana. Keep on hand a trail mix made with nuts, seeds, and a small amount of dried fruit.

- **Dessert.** Fruit, or a simple square of dark chocolate, preferably made with a natural sweetener.

STRATEGY 3. Use more fiber. Eating fiber helps keep your colon clean. A plant-based menu already contains some fiber, but there are simple ways to add more.

- Use brown rice, not white rice.

- Use whole-grain bread, not white bread.

- Eat bran muffins made with stevia or another non-sugar sweetener instead of pastry or croissants.

- Eat fresh fruit—a pear, or an apple, with skin.

- Eat a baked potato with the skin, or don't peel your mashed potatoes.

- Eat dried beans.

STRATEGY 4. Restrict your intake of animal foods.

- Eat red meat only occasionally, and try to keep the total amount of all meat you consume to no more than 15 percent of your total calories. (Avoid processed meats, such as hot dogs and cold cuts.)

- Reduce the portion size of meat when you do eat it. A portion should fit in the palm of your hand.

- You can use meat as a flavoring (for example, in a sauce) or side dish, not as an entrée.

- Substitute plant-based proteins for animal protein. For example, nuts and seeds (almonds, pecans, walnuts, pumpkin seeds, sesame seeds, sunflower seeds) can replace animal flesh.

- Choose leaner meats, such as chicken or turkey.

- Eat fish once or twice a week.

- Minimize dairy products, especially butter and cheese. Dairy contains lactose, which is milk sugar. Avoid cheese made with mold, such as Brie. When you do eat dairy, choose nonfat products, preferably fortified with omega-3 fatty acids.

- Eat four to six eggs a week.

STRATEGY 5. Choose good fats. Avocado oil, canola oil, olive oil, and sesame oil are unsaturated fats that decrease cancer risk. Avoid fats that increase cancer risk—saturated oils, such as those in whole-milk dairy products and red meat, and partially hydrogenated oils, which contain trans fatty acids, artificial fats created by adding hydrogen to vegetable oils to make them solid and extend their shelf life.

STRATEGY 6. Eat plenty of cancer-fighting foods.

- Boost your antioxidants. Best antioxidant sources are avocados, berries, green apples, lemons, and limes.

- Consume a wide range of brightly colored fruits and vegetables. The colors indicate that these foods are rich in phytochemicals, potent cancer-fighting and immune-boosting nutrients.

- Eat salmon, tuna, and flaxseeds; all are good sources of omega-3s.

- Use immune-boosting seasonings, such as basil, cilantro leaf, curry powder, ginger, garlic, rosemary, and turmeric.

- Eat some fruits and vegetables raw in order to get enzymes and the greatest amounts of vitamins and minerals.

STRATEGY 7. *Drink plenty of water, up to two quarts a day.* Keeping yourself well hydrated will increase your urine production and help eliminate toxins.

STRATEGY 8. *Maximize the cancer-fighting benefits of the food you eat.*

- Thoroughly wash all fruits and vegetables.

- Don't overcook. Steam vegetables in a small amount of water until just tender.

- Eat only organic food.

STRATEGY 9. *Avoid foods that impair your body's ability to heal.*

- Limit (or better yet, completely eliminate) fast foods, fried foods, and packaged foods.

- Avoid foods that contain fungus: mushrooms; fermented foods, such as pickles, sauerkraut, tempeh, and vinegar; and peanuts (which are all moldy). Fungus can contribute to cancer.

- Avoid sugar and any products containing it (read the labels—you'll be amazed at how many food products have been sweetened). Sugar is the *prime* growing medium for cancer and fungus. Use only stevia or xylitol as a sweetener. If you want to bake, use stevia.

STRATEGY 10. *Favor anti-angiogenic foods..* The foods in the list below boost the body's ability to suppress angiogenesis. (I include this strategy until the angiogenesis controversy is resolved.)

Apples, artichokes, blackberries, blueberries, bok choy, cherries, dark chocolate, garlic, ginseng, grapefruit, grapeseed oil, green tea, kale, lavender (in tea), lemons, licorice, maitake mushrooms, nutmeg, olive oil, oranges, parsley, pineapples, pomegranates, pumpkins, raspberries, red grapes, red wine, sea cucumber, soybeans, strawberries, tomato, tuna, and turmeric.

Note: These ten strategies are intended for cancer patients who don't have cachexia (wasting and weight loss). If you have cachexia, eat whatever food appeals to you—whatever you can get down—in order to sustain your weight.

FINAL THOUGHTS

I've waited until this late in the book to introduce the toxicity connection. But actually every single treatment, of any cancer patient, must *begin* by addressing this ninth connection. Why? Because it's far more difficult, sometimes even impossible, to address any of the other nine connections in an unclean, toxic body. The liver must be able to remove the toxins that are produced by the process of breaking down cancer cells and are accumulated through conventional treatments, especially chemo and radiation. To do this, the liver needs to work at full capacity, and for that it must be clean, just as an air conditioner needs a clean filter to function optimally. The intestine and colon must also be cleaned out, ready to handle all the toxic garbage that will be dumped into them.

Along with your detox, take your diet very seriously if you want to cure your cancer. Diet has two crucial functions—detoxifying and providing nutrients. It's a trite expression, but a true one, that you are what you eat. In fact, for anyone who doesn't have cancer and would like to prevent it, the best way to begin is diet.

Don't rely on anyone else to be the enforcer who makes you follow your anti-cancer diet. Take your fate in your own hands, and persevere. Although it may seem an exhausting effort to follow all the dietary strategies above, in the end it will pay off. And in any case, no one said it would be easy to survive the unsurvivable.

CHAPTER 10

– – – – –

Addressing the
Stress Connection

INITIAL THOUGHTS

As I see it, your desire to start a new treatment is a manifestation of your mind trying to help your body fight cancer. In this way, your mind creates a connection with your body. And I can't overstate the importance of this mind-body connection. It's a fact: your mind is the first line of defense against stress. And stress will not only make your cancer worse, but can literally kill you.

Indeed, stress is the worst enemy you can have when battling cancer, or any precancerous condition. People who have cancer must go on with their everyday lives, taking care of their job responsibilities, their family, figuring out their finances, paying bills, cooking, doing laundry, and loving their loved ones. For many, cancer isn't the only stress they face, it may not even be the main one. At the same time they contend with cancer, people may need to cope with other stressful events, such as loss of loved ones, divorce, loss of their job or health benefits, or difficulty paying the mortgage. Some of you may also encounter unsupportive attitudes from those same loved ones you rely on most. In particular, they may not support your decision to begin alternative treatment instead of continuing with conventional chemo and radiation.

Often oncologists suggest to advanced cancer patients that they visit a good hospice facility, to get familiar with the place and decide whether to go there when they're ready to die. Just imagine how much stress such a suggestion can cause. To me, it makes no sense. What's the rush? All it does is put the idea in the poor person's mind that he/she is going to die soon, instead of the more helpful idea of fighting the cancer and staying alive. This is the worst way to use the body-mind connection, and the best way to increase the person's stress level. I've seen many cases where this terrible suggestion winds up being the last straw because the body can take only so much stress. The physician's responsibility is to remove as much stress as possible, not increase it.

For all these reasons, the stress connection is a potent one that can have a powerful effect on your healing process. I've made it the tenth connection because it ties together all the others, but in fact you need to address it right from the start.

STRESS AND THE OTHER CANCER CONNECTIONS

Here are some of the physical effects of stress and their relation to the various cancer connections.

- Stress reduces the immune-system function (immune connection).

- Stress triggers the release of inflammatory cytokines and thereby increases inflammation (inflammation connection).

- Stress increases abdominal fat and insulin resistance (sugar, MID, and obesity connections).

- Stress increases the release of fats into the bloodstream, raises triglyceride levels, lowers good (HDL) cholesterol and raises bad (LDL) cholesterol (MID connection).

- Stress activates pathways that lead to the death of mitochondria and the loss of ATP production, and it decreases tissue oxygenation (oxygen connection).

- Stress increases depression and anxiety.

NEUROIMMUNOMODULATION AND PSYCHONEUROIMMUNOLOGY

Recent years have seen a great expansion in scientific explorations of the mind's ability to affect the body. One result of this work is neuroimmunomodulation (NIM), an area of research that studies how the nervous system and immune system interact and change (modulate) each other. Dr. Novera Herbert Spector, a scientist and physiologist who is considered the father of NIM, explained that you cannot stimulate one of these systems without a reaction from the other. As early as 1926, Serge Metalnikov, a scientist at the Pasteur Institute in Paris, conditioned guinea pigs to associate being scratched with an injection of bacteria. After that, the guinea pigs displayed the immune response in reaction to a scratch alone, even though no bacteria were present. In other words, the animals had an immune reaction purely to the stress created by the scratch.

Psychoneuroimmunology (PNI) is closely related to NIM. This term, which was coined by psychologist Robert Ader and immunologist Nicholas Cohen, describes a field of study that examines how the mind, nervous system, and various emotions all affect the immune system. They found that when rats were exposed to various forms of stress, the nervous system sent a signal stimulating release of stress hormones that suppressed the rats' immune systems. Other experiments demonstrated that stress increased tumor growth in mice. This research led to the development of the field of psycho-oncology, which is concerned with psychological factors and their effects on cancer. Most important, Ader's work triggered an increase in the use and study of a range of mind-body techniques as integrative cancer therapies.

In terms of my concept of the cancer connections, the main goal of psycho-oncology is, in essence, to address the stress connection. Understanding NIM and PNI allows you to appreciate the close and quite subtle relationships between stress and the other cancer connections in the list above. It is of the utmost importance that you break these relationships—sooner, rather than later.

STRESS RELIEF STRATEGIES

A study carried out at Ohio State University followed 227 women who had just received diagnoses of stage 2 or stage 3 breast cancer. Half the group participated in a psychological intervention program including relaxation training, positive ways to cope with stress and difficulties such as fatigue, methods to increase social support, and help with improving health through diet and exercise. After some years, sixty-two women had recurrences of breast cancer. Of these, the ones who had been in the stress-relief program were 59 percent less likely to die of their cancer. They had "significant emotional improvement and more favorable immune responses in the year following recurrence diagnosis," according to Barbara L. Andersen, the study's author.[1]

Even the experts at the Mayo Clinic, who are quite skeptical about integrative medicine, acknowledge that some alternative treatments "may provide some benefit." But don't get too excited. They're not suggesting IPT, oxidative therapies, Coley vaccine, or high doses of IV vitamin C. They simply describe a list of therapies that "may help you cope with signs and symptoms caused by cancer and cancer treatments."[2] For once, I'm in agreement with the Mayo Clinic, though for my own reason, because these therapies are instrumental in breaking the stress connection. A brief discussion of each therapy follows.

Acupuncture

An acupuncturist inserts very thin needles into specific points on the body, with the goal of restoring a healthy flow of the vital energy (called *qi* in Chinese). Some practitioners may twirl the needles or use a weak electric current that enhances their effects. Acupuncture is safe and extremely well researched. It has a synergistic effect with other integrative therapies. When used during surgery, radiotherapy, chemo, and immunotherapy, acupuncture can improve quality of life by:

- Alleviating stress and helping you relax;
- Decreasing nausea;
- Significantly reducing pain.

Aromatherapy

Aromatherapy uses aromatic essential oils to calm you and promote a sense of well-being. Some commonly used scents are rosemary, eucalyptus, lavender, ylang ylang, lemon, and geranium. The oils are applied to the skin during massage, added to bath water, or heated to release their fragrance into the air. Aromatherapy can alleviate pain, nausea, stress, and depression.

Massage Therapy

There are many forms of massage, which consists of manipulation of soft tissue by a trained practitioner, using the hands and sometimes forearms or elbows. Techniques range from deep, intense work, as in acupressure, fascial release (which works on the connective tissue to release tightness), or shiatsu (a traditional hands-on Japanese healing art), to light, gentle work, such as Reiki and Therapeutic Touch. Some massage therapists specialize in working with people being treated for cancer and know what techniques are appropriate at different stages.[3]

Massage can relieve pain, anxiety, fatigue, depression, and stress. It's also said to help eliminate toxins caused by chemo and radiation.

Exercise

The people at Mayo recommend gentle exercise, such as walking or swimming, as a way to reduce fatigue and stress and improve sleep. But exercise does more than that: it can break the inflammatory connection.

Inflammation is one of the body's natural protective mechanisms, but when it's chronic, it becomes destructive. Fortunately, exercise works like anti-inflammatory medicine. Muscle contraction releases myokines, a type of cytokine, that act to reduce inflammation. It seems that short-duration, high-intensity exercise, in which short bursts of all-out activity are interspersed with rest, is most effective for this purpose. This type of exercise can be adapted even for frail people.

In general, people with early-stage cancer can do intense exercise, while late-stage patients should do gentle exercise. Before engaging in any exercise program, speak to your physician, who can advise you about the type of exercise right for you.

Lifting Loads after Breast Cancer

A question for survivors of breast cancer is whether you need to avoid lifting heavy objects in order to decrease the risk of developing lymphedema after breast-cancer surgery that removed lymph nodes. Happily, the answer is no. A study conducted at the University of Pennsylvania School of Medicine followed 154 breast cancer patients with a history of having at least two lymph nodes removed in the previous five years. Half of these women participated in a supervised weight-lifting program. A year later, 17 percent of the women in the control group developed lymphedema, compared to only 11 percent of the women in the exercise group. Among women who had five or more lymph nodes removed, the benefit of exercise was even greater.[4]

In my opinion, it's just common sense that telling patients not to do any lifting after mastectomy is the same as telling people who have had a heart attack to stay in bed the rest of their life and never walk at all. My own experience demonstrates that some lifting is actually beneficial to *prevent* lymphedema, by maintaining a healthy flow of lymph.

Tai Chi and Yoga

Two techniques from Asia, tai chi and yoga, are excellent stress relievers.

Tai chi is an ancient Chinese martial art that involves gentle flowing movements and deep breathing, performed in a meditative way. It helps you become more agile and flexible, improves circulation, and relaxes both mind and body.

It's best to learn tai chi with an instructor, then you can continue the practice using books or videos. Its slow movements don't require great physical strength, and anyone can perform them easily. *Caution:* If any particular tai chi movement causes pain, don't do it.

Yoga is an ancient practice from India. It consists of a series of postures usually performed meditatively, with attention to breathing. The poses stretch, bend, and twist the body in a balanced way, and can be adapted for all levels of ability.

Styles of yoga range from highly aerobic to extremely gentle and restorative, so look for a class that suits your needs, and make sure you don't do any movements that cause pain. If a particular movement hurts you, the instructor will find alternative movements that don't. Some instructors specialize in yoga for cancer survivors. One place to find them is www.yogabear.com.

Using Your Mind to Heal

Since mind, body, and spirit are interconnected and affect each other, this connection is the basis of a number of therapeutic techniques that work with the mind to affect the body. Over the past few decades, scientists achieved a much greater understanding of how cancer develops, which led to the conventional trio of physical treatments. But the role the mind can play and its capacity to heal the body should not be underestimated.

This type of intervention focuses on the whole person. Using it will enable you to manage your symptoms much more easily and effectively, cope better with discomfort and distress, and most important, maintain hope. *And without hope, there is no hope.*

Meditation

Meditation is a state of focused awareness in which you place your attention on a specific image, sound, or positive idea and practice keeping it there. Deep breathing and deep relaxation exercises can also be done as forms of meditation.

Meditation can help relieve anxiety, pain, and stress. Ainslie Meares, an Australian psychiatrist, documented cases of cancer regression among patients who meditated. Meares worked with seventy-three patients who meditated for a minimum of twenty sessions. "Nearly all such patients should expect significant reduction of anxiety and depression, together with much less discomfort and pain," he reported.[5]

The best way to learn how to meditate is to find a class in guided meditation. Many clinics offer this training. There are also many resources on the Internet; for example, you can find scripts of guided meditations for cancer patients at www.healingcancernaturally.com.

Mindfulness-Based Stress Reduction is a program created by Dr. Jon Kabat-Zinn at the University of Massachusetts. Based on an ancient meditation technique and supported by twenty years of research, this eight-week program teaches how to work consciously and systematically with stress, pain, illness, and the challenges of everyday life. People who complete the course report decreased levels of pain and better ability to cope with any pain that remains, greater ability to cope with stress and relax, and diminished symptoms. To find a trained instructor in your area, go to www.umassmed.edu/cfm.

Affirmations

An affirmation is a direct, positive statement about yourself, your condition, and/or your ability to handle it. An example is, "I am in charge of my body and my mind. Therefore I am in charge of my cancer. It is not in charge of me."[6] Research by Dr. Bernie Siegel and others has shown that maintaining a positive mental state leads to better immune-system function, improved quality of life, even longer survival. Affirmations are an effective technique for helping shift into such a state.[7]

Imagery and Visualization

Throughout history, people have used their imaginations to help them heal. Envisioning your own well-being is the visual counterpart of verbal affirmations, and together these techniques are an important component of the overall healing process. A well-known technique that uses guided imagery is the Simonton method, developed by O. Carl Simonton and Stephanie Matthews-Simonton, and based on the principle that emotions and beliefs influence health and thus the body's ability to heal. In various exercises, patients visualize their bodies fighting off the cancer; for example, in one exercise you imagine small Pac-Man-type creatures attacking and destroying tumor cells. I strongly believe that all cancer patients will derive great benefit from using guided imagery in conjunction with medical treatments.

Hypnosis

Hypnosis is a trance-like state of concentrated yet relaxed attention in which the mind more easily takes in a suggestion because it is so focused. However, you always maintain control of your mind and can refuse any suggestion you don't like. During a hypnotherapy session, the practitioner helps you enter a hypnotic state by talking in a gentle voice, then puts a suggestion in your mind regarding its ability to heal your body. The therapist can also train you in self-hypnosis, so you have this technique available whenever you need it. Self-hypnosis CDs are also available.

Hypnotherapy can relax you, help prevent nausea and vomiting, relieve pain and fatigue, and help you sleep. It has a powerful ability to prepare you for surgery and other procedures so that you experience less trauma and recover more quickly. Anxiety is almost universal among cancer patients, who also often experience anger, helplessness, aloneness, guilt, alienation, hopelessness, low self-esteem, and loss. Hypnotherapy helps you cope with these emotions and achieve psychological harmony. And finally, both hypnosis and self-hypnosis can stimulate discoveries that lead to spiritual healing.

Music Therapy

"Music takes my mind and spirit to a place where cancer does not exist," a chemotherapy patient once wrote. I don't know anyone who isn't affected by music. Have you ever seen how, in the middle of a fight between spouses or parent and child, one party disappears to a private place and puts on his or her favorite music in order to calm down? Music can have a soothing effect on anyone, so it's no wonder that it can aid healing by shifting people out of worry, fear, anger, depression, or anxiety to a more positive state of mind.

Hospitals and medical offices now offer music therapy, often in conjunction with psychotherapy, guided imagery, hypnotherapy, or meditation. (Listening to a favorite piece of music is also an excellent meditation method.) A music therapy session is designed by the therapist according to the patient's needs and inclinations. You might listen to music, play an instrument, sing songs, even write lyrics. Music therapy can help relieve pain, control nausea and vomiting, relieve stress, ease insomnia, and provide a sense of well-being.

Relaxing music is helpful in preparing for surgery. It's also great to use during IPT, oxidative therapy, and other IV treatments.

Biofeedback

Biofeedback is a technique that trains your mind to control various body functions, such as heart rate, blood pressure, and muscle tension. The therapist uses an electronic device that monitors a body function. A beep or flashing light signals changes in your heart rate, for example. By focusing on altering this signal, you learn to control your heart rate with your mind. Biofeedback helps relieve pain and has also helped people regain urinary and bowel control after surgery.

MATCHING YOUR THERAPY TO YOUR SYMPTOMS

Here is a list of therapies that work best for different symptoms. You may find that it's most effective to use more than one therapy for each symptom.

TABLE 10.1	
Pain	Acupuncture, aromatherapy, hypnosis, meditation, massage, music therapy, biofeedback
Fatigue	Yoga, exercise, massage, acupuncture, music therapy
Nausea and vomiting	Acupuncture, hypnosis, aromatherapy, music therapy, meditation
Anxiety and depression	Hypnosis, meditation, massage, music therapy, yoga, tai chi
Stress	Music therapy, exercise, hypnosis, massage, meditation, yoga, tai chi, acupuncture, biofeedback
Sleep problems	Exercise, yoga, tai chi, meditation, music therapy

While using these therapies to address specific symptoms, you should also use guided imagery two or three times a day. And don't forget spirituality and the power of prayer. For many cancer patients, the positive effects of a prayer are a determining factor in their survival. So try praying.

FINAL THOUGHTS

Throughout the years that I've practiced integrative oncology, I've noticed one consistent phenomenon among my patients—those who fight their cancer aggressively have a much better chance of surviving. And those who decide at some point there's nothing more they can do are much less likely to survive.

I was stunned to discover that cancer patients whose oncologist informed them they had, say, a month to live—and who accepted this verdict—were gone in one month. By contrast, those who decided to fight it with everything they had—and more—lived much longer, and some survived. I know one woman who decided to leave the hospice facility where she had been sent to die within a week or two. She came home, began an aggressive integrative treatment program, and lived another five years.

Recently I called an oncologist who had treated one of my patients, to ask for information about her history. His response was, "Is she still alive?" Now I know he didn't wish in any way that she had died. He was just genuinely surprised that she hadn't. Many of my colleagues in integrative oncology will tell you similar stories—all examples of people applying their energy and determination to healing themselves, and excellent evidence of the crucial role of the mind-body connection.

Another good piece of advice—don't forget the power of humor. In his famous book, *Anatomy of an Illness,* Norman Cousins described how watching Marx Brothers movies helped him survive a life-threatening illness, when all his doctors expected him to die. Think positively, my friends, and don't forget to laugh.

Integrative and conventional oncology agree that alternative treatments providing stress relief are *beneficial.* However I would emphasize that they are more than beneficial. They are *essential,* since breaking the stress connection is just as important as breaking all the other nine connections.

Although the Mayo Clinic website I referred to above approves of stress-relief therapies, it warns that many other alternative treatments are unproven and actually dangerous. Now that you've read this entire book, you know what I think of that statement. So I'm not going to argue further with the experts of the prestigious Mayo Clinic about the safety of alternative treatments, especially when these treatments are compared with the many dangers of the conventional trio. I'd rather use laughter for my own healing.

- - - - -

The Cancer Connections— Blueprint for the Future

MY VERY FINAL THOUGHTS

I feel both happy and sad as I write these words. On one hand, I'm glad this book is nearly finished, but on the other, I feel attached to it, so I'm sorry it's ending.

All along, I've also felt very connected to you, my readers, and this feeling grew with each chapter. Though I don't actually know you personally, I *feel* that I do, because I sensed your presence all the time I was writing. Otherwise, who else was I talking to? So don't be surprised when I say I love you all and feel for you deeply. I'm also proud of you, since by reading this book you've shown your commitment to fighting this dreadful disease and never giving up.

The one important issue that remains for me to discuss is how to deal with either failure or success in your treatment. What do I mean by this? The course of your cancer can follow one of two scenarios. One is failure—test results that show either no change or a worsening of your condition. In that case, it's good to know that, if you try a therapy and it doesn't work, this does not spell failure. It's just one step toward making your program work for you. Some therapies work for some people; others work for other people. If a therapy fails you, don't feel like a failure yourself, just move on. I know for sure that by maintaining this attitude you'll give yourself a big boost. Sometimes when people start a new therapy and it doesn't work, they're ready to throw in the towel. Don't do that. That was only one attempt. Just go on to the next. Don't ever give up.

The other scenario is success: your pain is relieved, you feel much better, and the doctor may even announce that you're free of cancer. Often when cancer survivors hear this, they feel totally successful and decide that they're completely cured. But this is a serious misapprehension. To correct it, let me go back to the basics.

Just like asthma or diabetes, cancer is a *chronic degenerative disease.* You cannot cure such diseases, you can only control them. Most people, the moment their symptoms are gone, don't think much about whether their disease is cured or just controlled. But since my goal is for you to live a long, symptom-free life, I'm telling you that you must pay attention to this distinction. So let's assume that you're symptom-free, your tumor markers are pretty normal, and all the other tests are great. By no means should you relax and do nothing.

Instead, it's imperative that you continue addressing all the cancer connections in your body, in the different ways outlined in this book. Don't even consider stopping your treatment. And your first—probably only—treatment choice should be integrative oncology. It will serve all your needs and serve them well.

Choosing the right treatment options will require using your intellect and your common sense. Do research, ask questions, and speak with different doctors, patients, and support groups. Remember that integrative oncology offers you a far better chance of surviving and improving your quality of life than does conventional oncology. Most of you who read this book have probably come to this conclusion on your own.

The beauty of integrative oncology is manifold. First, it does not reject conventional treatments. In fact, one or more of the conventional trio is often a major part of an integrative approach, especially in the early stages of cancer. But both during and after any conventional treatment, you must also initiate alternative treatments. You need them right from the get-go.

A couple of days before writing this, I received a disturbing call from a woman named Mary. A year before, she had been diagnosed with early-stage breast cancer. It was a carcinoma in situ (localized), one of the less aggressive forms of breast cancer. After surgery and radiation, the oncologist told her she was completely cured, and she naturally took his word for it. Now she was calling to tell me that a more aggressive tumor had been discovered in her other breast. This sad story confirms two main principles this book has stressed, specifically that cancer develops in the body for twenty to thirty years before it can be detected, and that cancer is a chronic condition and must be treated as such.

So what was missing in the management of Mary's cancer? No doubt you can answer this question yourself. Because her cancer was only in an early stage and not aggressive at all, she did not think it necessary to use any form of integrative oncology. And her cancer proved her wrong. As I've explained, cancer is a disease not just of one organ—in her case, the breast—but of the whole body. So you can see why Mary would have done much better to apply the entire gamut of alternative treatments that this book has presented.

Integrative/alternative cancer therapies are diverse and many faceted. And this is the key to integrative oncology's effectiveness. At the risk of being redundant, let me reiterate: Cancer is a complicated disease, and a simple approach to it simply won't work. In most cases, the conventional *cut it, kill it, zap it* approach is not nearly sufficient, and now you know why. Cancer resides in an extremely complex place—the human body. And because of this complexity, both individual cancer cells and the tumor as a whole become involved in multiple interactions with a variety of body functions that can affect them either positively or negatively. The cancer cells and the tumor must interact with the body and respond to its requirements. That is why integration is the key concept of integrative oncology, and why the cancer connections are so important. They address all the facets of this complexity, and therefore they are the cornerstone of this book.

Integrative oncology is not just a convenient combination of different treatment modalities. It is an analytic system that examines different possible paths of cancer development and works to block these paths and, if possible, close them off completely. In fact I believe that the cancer connections will become the blueprint for a new systemic approach to integrative oncology. This approach, which has its birth in this book, can revolutionize all cancer treatment—even that of advanced cancers.

Ten cancer connections. The number ten carries a sense of mythic power (think of the ten commandments). The power of the ten cancer connections is that they provide a systematic approach to searching for the different causes that contribute to cancer. Breaking these connections, or even completely eliminating them, can greatly increase chances for survival. And the fact is that the improved survival seen in so many people after this type of treatment constitutes the great proof that integrative oncology and alternative cancer care are the way to tackle cancer in the twenty-first century. The logical—and humane—way to pursue the war on cancer, and ultimately win it, is the integrative way. I strongly believe that this integrative approach should become the mainstream approach in oncology.

But here I must insert a word of caution. You must be careful to pursue your integrative approach in a balanced way. It's unfortunate but true that greed and dishonesty can be present in the world of alternative treatment as well as in the conventional medical world. Look for an extremely knowledgeable, capable, and honest integrative physician whose entire focus is on your welfare. She or he should not be so wedded to one favored form of treatment that it is applied inappropriately. For each individual case, an integrative physician must carefully investigate both the conventional trio and a variety of alternative therapies. Alternative therapies may be nontoxic and harmless, but they may also not be right for you—and they may even be completely useless.

Integrative physicians realize that each person possesses different biochemical, emotional, physiological, and psychological characteristics that all together constitute his or her state of health. Integrative oncology pays attention to these individual distinctions. It respects the fact that making a diagnosis and decisions on treatment requires that the doctor take time to get to know a patient before applying her or his intuition and powers of observation to the person's case. Because integrative physicians do devote this time to their patients, they end up feeling extremely comfortable with these practitioners and appreciate being given sometimes quite gruesome and difficult information in a calm, tactful, and respectful way. This supportive bedside manner is also an important part of the integrative approach.

Despite its demonstrated success, the integrative approach remains a very difficult area of practice for the medical doctors, osteopaths, and naturopathic physicians who use it. The establishment's campaign against integrative/alternative cancer therapies and the practitioners who offer them continues. And instead of being acclaimed for seeking the best answer for cancer, integrative practitioners have been ridiculed, threatened, prosecuted, and even driven out of their profession and their countries. This closed-minded unwillingness to look honestly and thoroughly into alternative treatments is unbefitting a sophisticated, advanced country like the U.S. Americans on the whole are too intelligent, and too educated, for this nonsense.

And in fact, many people all over the world, including Americans, accept and understand the philosophy of natural medicine, and integrative oncology in particular. Americans' use of integrative/alternative medicine is increasing. According to a 2005 report sponsored by the National Institutes of Health and other government agencies, total visits to complementary/alternative medicine (CAM) providers each year now exceed those to primary-care physicians. Estimates of the prevalence of CAM use range from 30 to 62 percent of adults, depending on how CAM is defined.[1]

I believe that integrative oncology is presently in a transitional stage. In the past, I hardly ever got referrals from conventional oncologists, but now I'm getting more and more of them, some from physicians who have given up because they can do nothing more for their patients with the conventional trio. Some of these conventional doctors even suggest alternative treatments instead of sending their patients to hospice. For example, a very respected, traditional oncologist asked me to treat one of his patients with Iscador. My hope is that, in the twenty-first century, medicine will cease to be divided into two different types, conventional and alternative. Instead, there will just be one type: integrative medicine, with integrative oncology a part of it.

I'd like to make one last point in these very final thoughts. The significance of the ten cancer connections goes beyond your own personal case. That is why getting your oncologist involved would be of great benefit to others as well as yourself. Bring this book to your doctor (whether an integrative oncologist or a conventional one) to read. Maybe she or he will incorporate parts of it into your treatment program. A few such physicians might adopt its principles and in this way help many other people with cancer. The more the merrier. In fact just thinking about this makes me happy, since my greatest desire is that this book should become instrumental in everyone's personal journey to survive the unsurvivable. God bless you, God keep you, God save you.

References

Preface

1. Morgan G, et al. "The Contribution of Cytotoxic Chemotherapy to 5-Year Survival in Adult Malignancies." *Clinical Oncology (Royal College of Radiology)*. 16(8):549–660, Dec 2004.

Prologue—Cancer and Its Multiple Connections

1. Leaf, C. "Why We're Losing the War on Cancer, and How to Win It." *Fortune*. 78, Mar 22, 2004.

2. Apostolides AD, Apostolides, IK. "The United States Program on Cancer, 1975–2006: A Failure." *Townsend Letter*. 56, Oct 2010.

3. Taubes, G.. "Is Sugar Toxic?" *New York Times Magazine*. 8, Apr 17, 2011.

4. Peskin, B. "Cancer and Mitochondria Defects: New 21st Century Research." *Townsend Letter*. 89, Aug/Sept 2009.

5. "A Conversation With Polly Matzinger." *The New York Times,* http://www.nytimes.com/1998/06/16/science/conversation-with-polly-matzinger-blazing-unconventional-trail-new-theory.html?pagewanted=all&src=pm.

6. Hellmich, N. "Obesity Linked to Specific Cancers." *USA Today*. Nov. 5, 2009.

Chapter 1—Surgery, Chemo, Radiation

1. Formenti, SC. "Immunological Aspects of Local Radiotherapy: Clinical Relevance." *Johns Hopkins Discovery Medicine*. Feb 16, 2010. http://www.discoverymedicine.com/Silvia-C-Formenti/2010/02/16/immunological-aspects-of-local-radiotherapy-clinical-relevance/.

Chapter 2—Reduce Side Effects with Nutritional Strategies

1. Kennedy, DD, et al. "Low antioxidant vitamin intakes are associated with increases in adverse effects of chemotherapy in children with acute lymphoblastic leukemia." *American Journal of Clinical Nutrition*. 29(6):1029–1036, Jun 2004.

Cascinu S, et al. "Neuroprotective effect of reduced glutathione on oxaliplatin-based chemotherapy in advanced colorectal cancer." *Journal of Clinical Oncology*. 20(16):3478–3483, Aug 15, 2002.

2. Pathak, AK, et al. "Chemotherapy alone vs. chemotherapy plus high-dose multiple antioxidants in patients with advanced non-small-cell lung cancer." *Journal of the American College of Nutrition*. 24(1):16–21, 2005.

3. Lissoni P, et al. "Five-year survival in metastatic non-small-cell lung cancer patients treated with chemotherapy alone or chemotherapy and melatonin: a randomized trial." *Journal of Pineal Research.* 359:112–115, Aug 2003.

Chapter 3—Why Alternative Therapies Work

1. Upadhyay, J, Kesharwani, RK, Misra K. "Comparative study of antioxidants as cancer preventives through inhibition of HIF-1 alpha activity." *Bioinformation.* 4(6):233–236, 2009, http://www.bioin-formation.net/004/005300042009.pdf.

2. Murata, A, Morishige, F, Yamaguchi, H. "Prolongation of survival times of terminal cancer patients by administration of large doses of ascorbate." *International Journal for Vitamin and Nutrition Research Supplement.* 1982.

3. Chen, Q, et al. "Pharmacologic ascorbic acid concentrations selectively kill cancer cells: action as a pro-drug to deliver hydrogen peroxide to tissues." *Proceedings of the National Academy of Sciences U S A.* 102(38):13604–13609, Sep 20; 2005. http://www.ncbi.nlm.nih.gov/pubmed/16157892.

4. Moss, RW. "Intriguing New Anticancer Compound From East Europe." http://www.ralphmoss .com/ukrain.html.

5. Robey, IF, et al. "Bicarbonate Increases Tumor pH and Inhibits Spontaneous Metastases." *Cancer Research.* 69:(6), Mar 15, 2009.

Chapter 4—Insulin Potentiation Therapy

1. My summary of Annie Brandt's story and all the quotes in this section come from her own account: Annie Brandt, "How IPT Saved My Life," in *The Kinder, Gentler Cancer Treatment: Insulin Potentiation Targeted LowDose Therapy.* BookSurge Publishing. 7, 2009.

2. Lasalvia-Prisco, E, et al. "Insulin-induced enhancement of antitumoral response to methotrexate in breast cancer patients." *Cancer Chemotherapy and Pharmacology.* 53(3):220–224, Mar 2004. Epub Dec 4, 2003.

Chapter 5—Immunotherapy and Cancer Vaccines

1. Leaf, C. "Why We're Losing the War on Cancer: And How To Win It." *Fortune.* 85, Mar 22, 2004.

2. As described by Hobohm, U. "Fever and cancer in perspective." *Cancer Immunology and Immunotherapy.* 50: 391–396, 2001.

3. Marshall, J. "Filthy Healthy: The Cancer Hygiene Hypothesis." *The New Scientist,* 197:2638, 34–37, January 12, 2008.

4. Dreifus, C. "A Conversation With Polly Matzinger," *The New York Times,* June 16, 1998, http://www.nytimes.com/1998/06/16/science/conversation-with-polly-matzinger-blazing-unconventional-trail-new-theory.html?pagewanted=all&src=pm

5. Matzinger, P. "The Four Ds of the Danger Model: Distress, Damage, Destruction, and Death." In John C. Marshall and Jonathan Cohen, *Immune Response in the Critically Ill.* Springer-Verlag. 9, 2002.

6. Dermatology|Yale School of Medicine, "Transimmunization," n.d., http://medicine.yale.edu/dermatology/clinical/medderm/transimmunization/index.aspx

Chapter 6—Oxidative Therapies

1. Zimran, A, et al. "Effect of ozone on red blood cell enzymes and intermediates." *Acta Haematologica.* 102(3):148–151, 2000.

2. Bocci, V, et al. "The ozone paradox: ozone is a strong oxidant as well as a medical drug." *Medical Care Research and Review.* 29(4):646–682, Jul 2009.

3. Clavo, B, et al. "Adjuvant Ozonetherapy in Advanced Head and Neck Tumors: A Comparative Study." published online Oct 16, 2004. http://www.ncbi.nlm.nih.gov/pmc/articles/PMC538509/?tool=pubmed.

4. Clavo, B, et al. "Intravesical ozone therapy for progressive radiation-induced hematuria." *Journal of Alternative and Complementary Medicine.* (3):539–541, Jun11, 2005.

5. Kontorschikova, CN, Alaysova, AV, Terentiev, IG. "Ozone therapy in a Complex Treatment of Breast Cancer." In: Proceedings of the 15th Ozone World Congress, 11th–15th Sept 2001, Medical Therapy Conference (IOA 2001, Ed.). Ealing, London, UK: *Speedprint Macmedia Ltd,* 2001.

6. Van den Brenk, HA, Madigan, JP, Kerr, RC. "An analysis of the progression and development of metastases in patients receiving x-radiation in hyperbaric oxygen." *Clinical Radiology.* (1):54–61, Jan 18, 1967.

7. Casanovas, O, Hicklin, DJ, Bergers, G, et al. "Drug resistance by evasion of antiangiogenic targeting of VEGF signaling in late-stage pancreatic islet tumors." *Cancer Cell.* 8(4):299–309, Oct 2005.

Pàez-Ribes, M, Allen, E, Hudock, J, et al."Antiangiogenic therapy elicits malignant progression of tumors to increased local invasion and distant metastasis." *Cancer Cell.* 15(3):220–231, 2009.

8. "Starve a Tumor, or Feed a Tumor?" University of Rochester Medical Center, http://www.urmc.rochester.edu/news/story/index.cfm?id=375.

Chapter 7—Off-Label Use of Drugs

1. Makman, MH. "Morphine receptors in immunocytes and neurons." *Advances in Neuroimmunology.* 4(2):69–82, 1992.

2. Ballantyne, JC, Mao, J. "Opioid Therapy for Chronic Pain." *New England Journal of Medicine.* 349:1943–1953, Nov 13, 2003.

3. "Metformin for Cancer: Off-label Cancer Treatments," n.d., http://cancerx.wordpress.com/2008/10/26/off-label-metformin-for-cancer/.

4. Evans, JMM, et al. "Metformin and reduced risk of cancer in diabetic patients." *British Medical Journal.* 330(7503):1304–1305, June 4; 2005.

5. Armitage, JO, Sidney, RD. "Antitumor effect of cimetidine." *The Lancet.* 1(8121):882–883, 1979.

6. "Cimetidine for Cancer," n.d., http://cancerx.wordpress.com/?s=cimetidine.

7. Chen, S, et al. "Celecoxib promotes c-FLIP degradation through Akt-independent inhibition of GSK3." *Cancer Research.* Aug 25, 2011.

8. Arber, N, et al. "Five-year analysis of the prevention of colorectal sporadic adenomatous polyps trial." *American Journal of Gastroenterology.* 106(6):1135–1146, Jun 2011. Epub Apr 19, 2011.

9. http://cancerx.wordpress.com/2009/02/08/statins-for-cancer/.

10. "Medicor Cancer Centre's Observational DCA Treatment Data." http://www.medicorcancer.com/archiveData_12-12-07.html.

11. Sun T, et al. "Doxycycline inhibits the adhesion and migration of melanoma cells by inhibiting the expression and phosphorylation of focal adhesion kinase (FAK)." *Cancer Letters.* 285(2):141–150, Nov 28, 2009. Epub May 30, 2009.

12. Chang, JG, et al. "Small Molecule Amiloride Modulates Oncogenic RNA Alternative Splicing to Devitalize Human Cancer Cells." PLoS One. 6(6):2011. e18643. Published online http://www.ncbi.nlm.nih.gov/pmc/articles/PMC3111415, June 9, 2011.

13. Sparks, RL, et al. "Effects of Amiloride on Tumor Growth and Intracellular Element Content of Tumor Cells *in Vivo.*" *Cancer Research.* 43: 73, Jan 1983.

14. http://cancerx.wordpress.com/2008/11/10/dipyridamole-for-cancer/.

15. The European Stroke Prevention Study (ESPS). Principal end-points. The ESPS Group. *The Lancet.* 8572(2):1351–1354, Dec 12; 1987.

16. http://cancerx.wordpress.com/2008/11/10/dipyridamole-for-cancer/.

17. http://cancerx.wordpress.com/2008/11/24/disulfiram-antabuse-for-cancer.

18. Sukhdev, SB, et al. "Disulfiram inhibits activating transcription factor/cyclic AMP-responsive element binding protein and human melanoma growth in a metal-dependent manner in vitro, in mice and in a patient with metastatic disease." *Molecular Cancer Therapeutics.* 3:1049, Sept 2004. http://mct.aacrjournals.org/content/3/9/1049.long.

19. Gills, JJ, et al. "Nelfinavir, A lead HIV protease inhibitor, is a broad-spectrum, anticancer agent that induces endoplasmic reticulum stress, autophagy, and apoptosis in vitro and in vivo." *Clinical Cancer Research.* 13(17):5183–5194, Sep 1, 2007.

20. Gupta, AK, et al. "HIV protease inhibitors block Akt signaling and radiosensitize tumor cells both in vitro and in vivo." *Cancer Research.* 65(18):8256–8265, Sep 15, 2005.

21. Brunner, TB, et al. "Phase I trial of the human immunodeficiency virus protease inhibitor nelfinavir and chemoradiation for locally advanced pancreatic cancer." *Journal of Clinical Oncology.* 26(16):2699–2706, Jun 1, 2008.

Chapter 8—Natural Substances Fight Cancer

1. Oberlies, NH, et al. "Structure-activity relationships of diverse Annonaceous acetogenins against multidrug-resistant human mammary adenocarcinoma (MCF-7/Adr) cells." *Cancer Letters.* 115: 73–79, 1997.

2. www.facr.org/pdf/information-packet-updated.pdf.

3. "Mounting Evidence Shows Red Wine Antioxidant Kills Cancer." http://www.urmc.rochester.edu/news/story/index.cfm?id=1934.

4. Choi, H, et al. "Curcumin inhibits hypoxia-inducible factor-1." *Molecular Pharmacology.* 70(5):1064–1071, 2006.

5. Friedman, M, et al. "Structure-activity relationships of tea compounds against human cancer cells." *Journal of Agricultural and Food Chemistry.* 55(2):243–253, Jan 24, 2007.

6. Shanafelt, TD, et al. "Phase II trial of daily, oral green tea extract in patients with asymptomatic, Rai stage 0-II chronic lymphocytic leukemia (CLL)." *Journal of Clinical Oncology.* 28:15s (suppl; abstr 6522), 2010.

7. Tyagi A, et al. "Silibinin causes cell cycle arrest and apoptosis in human bladder transitional cell carcinoma cells by regulating CDKI-CDK-cyclin cascade, and caspase 3 and PARP cleavages." *Carcinogenesis.* (9):1711–1720, Sep 25, 2004. Epub Apr 29, 2004.

8. Folkers, K, et al. "The activities of coenzyme Q_{10} and vitamin B_6 for immune responses." *Biochemical and Biophysical Research Communications.* 192:241–245, Apr 15, 1993.

Lockwood, K, et al. "Partial and complete regression of breast cancer in patients in relation to dosage of coenzyme Q_{10}." *Biochemical and Biophysical Research Communications.* 199:1504–1508, Mar 30, 1994.

9. Singh, NP, Lai, H. "Selective toxicity of dihydroartemisinin and holotransferrin toward human breast cancer cells." *Life Sciences.* 70:49–56, 2001.

10. Ohgami, Y, et al. "Effect of hyperbaric oxygen on the anti-cancer effect of artemisinin on molt-4 human leukemia cells." *Anti-Cancer Research.* 30(11):4467–4470, Nov 2010. http://www.washington.edu/news/articles/high-dose-of-oxygen-enhances-natural-cancer-treatment.

11. Yan, J, Katz, A. "PectaSol-C Modified Citrus Pectin Induces Apoptosis and Inhibition of Proliferation in Human and Mouse Androgen-Dependent and Independent Prostate Cancer Cells." *Integrative Cancer Therapies.* 9(2):197–203. Jun 2010.

12. Yang, P, et al. "Zyflamend reduces LTB4 formation and prevents oral carcinogenesis in a 7,12-dimethylbenz[alpha]anthracene (DMBA)-induced hamster cheek pouch model." *Carcinogenesis.* 29(11):2182–2189; Nov 2008.

Yang, P, et al. "Zyflamend-mediated inhibition of human prostate cancer PC3 cell proliferation: effects on 12-LOX and Rb protein phosphorylation." *Cancer Biology & Therapy.* 6(2):228–236, Feb 2007. Epub Feb 25, 2007.

13. "Pepper Component Hot Enough To Trigger Suicide In Prostate Cancer Cells." http://cedars-sinai.edu/About-Us/News/News-Releases-2006/Pepper-Component-Hot-Enough-To-Trigger-Suicide-In-Prostate-Cancer-Cells-.aspx.

14. Khan, A, et al. "Cinnamon improves glucose and lipids of people with type 2 diabetes." *Diabetes Care.* 26(12):3215–3218, Dec 2003.

15. Wutzke, KD, Lorenz, H. "The Effect of l-Carnitine on Fat Oxidation, Protein Turnover, and Body Composition in Slightly Overweight Subjects." *Metabolism.* 53(8):1002–1006, 2004.

16. Reda, E, et al. "The Carnitine System and Body Composition." *Acta Diabetologica.* 40:106–113, 2003.

17. Cavaliere, H, Medeiros-Neto, G. "The anorectic effect of increasing doses of L-tryptophan in obese patients." *Eating and Weight Disorders.* 2(4):211–215, Dec 1997.

Chapter 9—Toxins and How to Get Rid of Them

1. Layton, L. "U.S. facing 'grievous harm' from chemicals in air, food, water, panel says." *Washington Post,* May 7, 2010. http://www.washingtonpost.com/wp-dyn/content/article/2010/05/06/AR20100 50603813.html.

2. *Cancer and the Environment: What You Need to Know, What You Can Do.* 1. http://www .cancer.gov/newscenter/Cancer-and-the-Environment.

3. Kross, B, et al. "Proportional mortality study of golf course superintendents." *American Journal of Industrial Medicine.* 29:501–506, 1996.

4. Rapp, D. *Our Toxic World: A Wake Up Call,* Environmental Research Foundation. 234, 2003.

5. National Research Council, Board on Agriculture, Committee on Scientific and Regulatory Issues Underlying Pesticide Use Patterns and Agricultural Innovation, "Regulating Pesticides in Food: The Delaney Paradox." *National Academy Press.* 4, 1967.

6. Cantor, K, Silberman, W. "Mortality among aerial pesticide applicators and flight instructors: follow-up from 1965–1988." *American Journal of Industrial Medicine*. 36(2) 239–247, 1999.

7. Barker, DJP, et al. "Fetal origins of adult diseases." *European Journal of Epidemiology*. 18(8):733–736, 2003.

8. Nash, MJ. "The Enemy Within." *Time*. Sept 18, 1996.

9. Doyle, R. *Scientific American*, Oct. 1995. http://cool.conservation-us.org/waac/wn/wn18/wn18-1/wn18-105.html.

10. Burton Goldberg Group. *Alternative Medicine: The Definitive Guide*. Tiburon, CA: Future Medicine Publishing. 186, 1995.

11. Maugh, TH, II. "Experts Downplay Cancer Risk of Chlorinated Water." *Los Angeles Times*. July 2, 1992. http://articles.latimes.com/1992-07-02/local/me-1814_1_drinking-water.

12. National Cancer Institute. "Fluoridated Water: Questions and Answers." http://www.cancer.gov/cancertopics/factsheet/Risk/fluoridated-water#r5.

13. Steinman, D. *Diet for a Poisoned Planet*. New York, NY: Ballantine. 265, 1992.

14. Feychting, M, Ahlbom, A. "Childhood Leukemia and Residental Exposure to Weak Extremely Low Frequency Magnetic Fields." *Environmental Health Perspectives* (Suppl 2), 59–62, 1995.
      Savitz, DA. "Overview of Epidemiologic Research on Electric and Magnetic Fields and Cancer." *American Industrial Hygiene Association Journal*. 54:4, 197–204, 1993. Epub Feb 25, 2007.

15. Savitz, DA, Loomis, DP. "Magnetic Field Exposure in Relation to Leukemia and Brain Cancer Mortality Among Electric Utility Workers." *American Journal of Epidemiology*. 141:2:123–134, 1995.
      Loomis, DP, Savitz, DA. "Mortality from Brain Cancer and Leukemia among Electrical Workers." *British Journal of Industrial Medicine*. 47(9):633–638, 1990. Epub Feb 25, 2007.

Chapter 10—Addressing the Stress Connection

1. http://clincancerres.aacrjournals.org/content/early/2010/06/01/1078-0432.CCR-10-0278.
   http://www.businessweek.com/print/lifestyle/content/healthday/639923.html.

2. http://www.mayoclinic.com/health/cancer-treatment/CM00002.

3. http://www.medicinehands.com http://www.massagetherapy.com/articles/index.php?article_id=142.

4. Cox, L. "Weight lifting OK for breast cancer survivors." http://www.msnbc.msn.com/id/40577341/ns/health-cancer/t/weight-lifting-ok-breast-cancer-survivors/#.TrrNi1Y1Snk.

5. Lerner, M. In *Choices in Healing: Integrating the Best of Conventional and Complementary Approaches to Cancer*. Cambridge, MA: MIT Press. 151, 1994.

6. Cancer affirmations: http://www.lexpages.com/SGN/paschal/cancerbeliefs.html.

7. http://www.healingcancernaturally.com/power-of-thought-to-heal-1.html.

Conclusion

1. Committee on the Use of Complementary and Alternative Medicine by the American Public, *Complementary and Alternative Medicine in the United States*. Washington, D.C., National Academies Press. 10, 2005. Available free at http://www.nap.edu/openbook.php?record_id=11182&page=1.

Resources

American Holistic Medical Foundation
27629 Chagrin Blvd., Suite 213
Woodmere, OH 44122
Ph: 216-292-6644
Email: info@holisticmedicine.org
Website: http://www.holisticmedicine.org

On the AHMF website you can search for individual providers and for integrative medicine centers affiliated with universities throughout the U.S.; click on "Holistic Resources" under "Holistic Medicine." The website includes many other informational resources as well.

Best Answer for Cancer Foundation Patient Survivor Center
8127 Mesa, B-206 #213
Austin, TX 78759
Ph: 512-342-8181
Email: annie@bestanswerforcancer.org
Website: www.bestanswerforcancer.org/patientsurvivor-center

This website features a forum that includes a chat room and a message board.

Cancer Decisions
PO Box 1076
Lemont, PA 16851
Ph: 800-980-1234
Ph outside USA: 814-238-3367
Website: http://cancerdecisions.com

This site of medical writer Ralph W. Moss, Ph.D., offers information about alternative/integrative treatments, a newsletter, phone consultations, and up-to-date reports on specific types of cancer written by Moss.

Center for Mindfulness in Medicine, Health Care, and Society
University of Massachusetts Medical School
55 Lake Avenue North
Worcester, MA 01655
Ph: 508-856-2656
Email: mindfulness@umassmed.edu
Website: http://www.umassmed.edu/cfm/home/index.aspx
The Center pioneered the development of Mindfulness-Based Stress Reduction.
To find an MBSR instructor in your area, click on "The Stress Reduction Program."

Healing Cancer Naturally • Website: www.healingcancernaturally.com
Website includes scripts of guided meditations for people who have cancer.

IPT for Cancer • Website: www.iptforcancer.com
On this website, sponsored by Annie Brandt's Best Answer for Cancer Foundation,
you can locate IPT practitioners.

Pavel I. Yutsis, M.D.
3849 Nostrand Avenue
Brooklyn , NY 11235
Ph: 718-368-9555
Email: lifex3849@aol.com
Website: www.dr.yutsis.com

The Institute for Healthy Aging
Mark A. Rosenberg, M.D., Medical Director
4800 North Federal Highway
Suite B103
Boca Raton, FL 33431
Ph: 561-939-3898
Website: www.antiagemed.com

The institute offers individualized treatments to slow and even reverse the aging
process, weight loss programs, and alternative cancer treatments that complement
conventional cancer therapy.

Yoga Bear
Website: www.yogabear.com

This nonprofit connects cancer survivors with free therapeutic and restorative yoga
classes taught by practitioners who specialize in working with cancer survivors,
as well as a support community.

Index

About the Authors

Pavel I Yutsis, M.D., is an integrative/complementary physician who is board certified in chelation therapy, oxidative medicine, and naturopathic medicine, and is a Fellow in Integrative Cancer Therapy of the American Academy of Anti-Aging Medicine. Dr. Yutsis is well known in the medical community for his cutting-edge work in nutritional therapies, including metabolic immunodepression. In addition to the American Academy of Anti-Aging Medicine, he is a member of the American Academy of Environmental Medicine, the American Academy of Preventive Medicine, the American College for Advancement in Medicine, and the Broda Barnes, M.D., Research Foundation. He has written numerous articles for medical journals and is the author of several books, including *Oxygen To The Rescue* (also published by Basic Health Publications), *The Downhill Syndrome,* and *Why Can't I Remember? Reversing Normal Memory Loss.* He lives and has his integrative medical practice in Brooklyn, New York.

Stephanie Golden is a medical writer, journalist, and nonfiction author. She wrote *Slaying the Mermaid: Women and the Culture of Sacrifice; The Women Outside: Meanings and Myths of Homelessness* (a finalist for the Robert F. Kennedy Book Award), and *Compulsive Behavior,* a book for teenagers on obsessive-compulsive disorder. She has also co-authored six books, including *Under the Mask: A Guide to Feeling Secure and Comfortable during Anesthesia and Surgery* with James E. Cottrell, M.D. She lives and works in Brooklyn, New York.